OPHTHALMOLOGY MONOGRAPHS 1

Retinal Detachment

Principles and Practice

SECOND EDITION

American Academy of Ophthalmology
655 Beach Street
P.O. Box 7424
San Francisco, CA 94120-7424

Design and Production
Christy Butterfield Design

This continuing medical education activity was planned and produced in accordance with the Essentials of the Accreditation Council for Continuing Medical Education.

OPHTHALMOLOGY MONOGRAPHS 1

Retinal Detachment

Principles and Practice

SECOND EDITION

George F. Hilton, MD

Edward B. McLean, MD

Daniel A. Brinton, MD

AMERICAN ACADEMY OF OPHTHALMOLOGY

LEO
Lifelong Education for the Ophthalmologist

Library of Congress Cataloging-in-Publication Data

Hilton, George F.
Retinal detachment : principles and practice / George F. Hilton, Edward B. McLean, Daniel A. Brinton. — 2nd ed.
p. cm. — (Ophthalmology monographs ; 1)
Rev. ed. of: Retinal detachment. 5th ed. [i.e. 1st ed.]. 1989.
Includes bibliographical references and index.
ISBN (invalid) 1-65055-028-7
1. Retinal detachment. 2. Retinal detachment—Surgery.
I. McLean, Edward B., 1935– . II. Brinton, Daniel A., 1955– .
III. Title. IV. Series.
[DNLM: 1. Retinal Detachment. W1 OP372L v. 1 1995 / WW 270 H656r 1995]
RE603.H543 1995
617.7'3—dc20
DNLM/DLC 94-43382
for Library of Congress CIP

99 98 97 96 95 5 4 3 2 1

Contents

Preface

This monograph was written on assignment from the American Academy of Ophthalmology. Rather than document each point, we have chosen to present the material in a didactic fashion without specific references to the literature. A list of Suggested Readings is included at the end of each chapter for those who would like to pursue further research.

The work is based on a review of the literature and on our personal experience. We have attempted to acknowledge controversy where it exists and to present alternative points of view. The monograph is sufficiently brief to encourage cover-to-cover reading, but it is organized in discrete sections and has a detailed table of contents and an index to facilitate locating specific information. The book is not an all-inclusive treatise; rather, it is intended as an introduction to retinal detachment for the graduate student in ophthalmology. It may also serve the practicing ophthalmologist as a concise review of the subject or as a reference source.

We are pleased to include as an appendix the classic article "The Technique of Binocular Indirect Ophthalmoscopy" written by Morton L. Rosenthal, MD, and illustrated by Seymour Fradin, MD. The treatise should be studied carefully by anyone who aspires to cure patients afflicted with detachment of the retina.

The many changes from the first edition of this monograph, published in 1989, include

- Contemporary guidelines for managing breaks without retinal detachment
- An innovative six-point "menu" for managing detachment
- New insights into the critical problem of case selection for pneumatic retinopexy
- Current information on using the episcleral gelatin buckle for children
- Commentary on the two classifications of proliferative vitreoretinopathy
- Comparative results of scleral buckling versus pneumatic retinopexy
- Updated suggested readings

The educational objectives of the monograph are to

- Provide a historical review of the diagnosis and treatment of retinal detachment
- Offer contemporary information on the subject of retinal detachment
- Afford ophthalmologists the opportunity to evaluate their knowledge of the basic and clinical aspects of retinal detachment
- Supply a reference for managing retinal detachment patients in the office, clinic, or hospital
- Publish an up-to-date guide to the relevant literature on retinal detachment

The treatment of retinal detachment is continually changing, and an accelerated rate of change in the future is anticipated. We would be most grateful to any reader who would take the time to inform us of any errors in the monograph, either of commission or omission.

George F. Hilton, MD
Edward B. McLean, MD
Daniel A. Brinton, MD

CHAPTER 1

Historical Introduction

The evolution of the retinal reattachment operation is one of the most remarkable chapters in the history of ophthalmology. Gonin's operation for repair of the detached retina ranks with Daviel's cataract extraction, von Graefe's peripheral iridectomy, and Machemer's vitrectomy as one of the four greatest surgical treatments for blindness. Gonin's landmark work and influence serve as the focus around which the following historical review of the diagnosis and treatment of retinal detachment is organized (Figure 1-1).

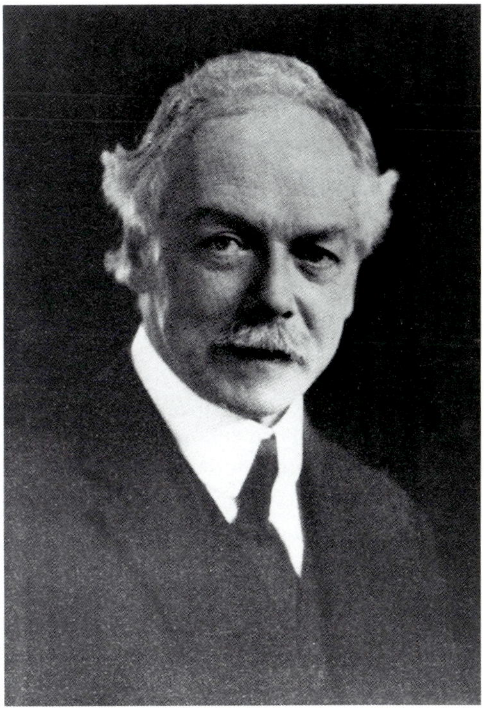

Figure 1-1 *Jules Gonin, MD, 1870–1935, father of retinal detachment surgery.*
Reproduced with permission from Duke-Elder S, ed: Diseases of the Retina, *vol X of* System of Ophthalmology. *St Louis: CV Mosby Co; 1967.*

1-1

THE PRE–GONIN PERIOD

The entity of retinal detachment was recognized early in the eighteenth century by de Saint-Yves, who reported the gross pathologic examination of an eye with a detached retina. But the first clinical description did not appear until almost a century later, in 1817, when Beer reported his detection of a retinal detachment in a patient. This detachment must have been immediately posterior to the lens, because he was able to observe it without the benefit of an ophthalmoscope.

Von Helmholtz's invention of the direct ophthalmoscope in 1851 was a giant step forward in diagnostic technique, and a rapid succession of ophthalmoscopic observations of detachments followed shortly thereafter. In the same year, Coccius reported the ophthalmoscopic detection of breaks in the retina.

Von Graefe theorized in 1858 that retinal detachment is caused by a serous effusion from the choroid into the subretinal space. When he observed a retinal break, he assumed that it was secondary to the detachment and represented the eye's attempt to cure itself. He supposed that, with the development of a break, the subretinal fluid could pass from the subretinal space into the vitreous cavity. With this conviction, he attempted to treat detachments with deliberate incision of the retina, but of course this therapeutic approach was destined to fail.

Girard-Teulon invented the reflecting binocular indirect ophthalmoscope in 1861. This potentially important contribution was generally overlooked by the profession. Therefore, more than 80 years transpired before Schepens developed the self-luminous binocular indirect ophthalmoscope.

In 1869 Iwanoff became the first person to describe the entity of posterior vitreous detachment, which is now recognized as an essential prerequisite to the development of most retinal detachments. The following year de Wecker proposed a point of view opposite von Graefe's, suggesting that the retinal break causes the detachment due to the resultant passage of fluid vitreous from the vitreous cavity through the break into the subretinal space. Unfortunately, his accurate interpretation fell on deaf ears. In 1882 Leber reported his observation of retinal breaks in 14 of 27 retinal detachments, and he correctly inferred the role of vitreous traction in the pathogenesis of breaks. Later in his career, Leber changed his mind, partly clouding his contribution to the field. In 1889 Deutschmann treated a detachment by closing the retinal break with ignipuncture. However, the value of this procedure was not appreciated at the time, and it was set aside for several decades.

1-2

THE GONIN PERIOD

Jules Gonin (1870–1935) was born in Lausanne, Switzerland, where he was also educated and pursued his brilliant career. He graduated from the University of Lausanne Medical School in 1894, spent 1 year training in pathology, and then entered ophthalmic training under the direction of Professor Marc Dufour, a former assistant of von Graefe. Dufour invited Gonin, in 1904, to collaborate with him in updating the chapter on diseases of the retina and optic nerve in the *French Encyclopedia of Ophthalmology*. As Gonin pursued this assignment, his attention was focused on the treatment of retinal detachment, which at the time was viewed with great pessimism. He was particularly interested in the works of Leber and became convinced of the causal role of retinal breaks in the pathogenesis of retinal detachment.

Thereafter, Gonin devoted many years to study in the laboratory and the clinic, producing many scientific papers on a variety of subjects. He was instrumental in the establishment of the Swiss Ophthalmological Society. In 1918 he was appointed to the Chair of Ophthalmology at the University of Lausanne and took on the position of chief surgeon at the eye hospital.

Resurrecting Deutschmann's surgical approach, Gonin treated retinal breaks with a red-hot searing probe. (He obtained the probe, which was manufactured for burning designs in wood, at a toy store.) Gonin first reported his results to the French Ophthalmological Society in 1923 and to the Heidelberg Congress in 1925, but the great therapeutic potential described in these initial reports was generally overlooked by his colleagues. Later, widespread interest was aroused by a paper he presented at the 1929 International Congress of Ophthalmology in Amsterdam, in which he reported the surgical cure of 20 of 30 cases of retinal detachment that had existed for 3 weeks or less. However, he reported a cure of only 15 of 35 detachments persistent for more than 3 months.

To Gonin goes the credit not only for developing his operation, but also for promoting and disseminating the new treatment through the publication of 34 papers in Belgian, German, British, American, Swiss, and French journals. In each he emphasized the essential role of retinal breaks and the necessity of closing them with his searing method, ignipuncture.

Ophthalmologists from all over the world visited Lausanne, and Gonin's operation was first introduced across the Atlantic by Schoenberg, who performed it in the United States in 1929. Pischel was later instrumental in its popularization in the United States. In 1934 Gonin published his classic text, *Retinal Detachment.*

A condition that previously had been a uniform cause of blindness responded to Gonin's operation in about 60% of cases. His memory is perpetuated by the Club Jules Gonin, an international society of retinal surgeons, and a commemorative plaque is now prominently displayed on Avenue Jules Gonin in Lausanne.

1-3

THE POST–GONIN PERIOD

Gonin's procedure was markedly improved in the early 1930s when Weve and Larsson independently developed the use of diathermy in place of the red-hot searing technique. In 1933 Lindner approached the problem of retinal detachment by attempting to reduce the volume of the globe and shorten the axial length with full-thickness scleral resection, an adaptation of the scleral resection developed by Müller. The first description of scleral buckling was recorded in 1937 by Jess, but this brief mention in the literature was not pursued, and the ophthalmic world had to wait another 12 years for the full development of scleral buckling.

Rosengren's popularization of the use of intravitreal air injection for the closure of retinal breaks, which he developed in 1938, reflected the attention directed at the time toward bringing the choroid against detached retinal breaks by internal as well as external pressure.

In 1945 Schepens modified and developed the modern binocular indirect ophthalmoscope. Now widely used, Schepens' contribution has been augmented by the use of scleral indentation (scleral "depression"), a technique originally introduced by Trantas. With this technique, the periphery of the retina can be brought more clearly into view and, more importantly, peripheral lesions can be viewed in dynamic profile as they are gently massaged by the scleral indentor.

A great debt is owed Custodis for the development in 1949 of scleral buckling. He used a polyviol plomb, which was sutured to the surface of the globe and thereby created a prominent segmental scleral buckle. Moreover, he made the remarkable contribution of demonstrating that many retinal detachments can be cured without actually closing the retinal break. He proved that if a scleral indentation was produced beneath the retinal break, in most cases the fluid would subsequently be absorbed, even if the break had not been closed at the time of surgery. Just how this buckle promotes the absorption of subretinal fluid is still not fully understood.

In 1949 Shapland supplanted Lindner's full-thickness resection with a lamellar scleral resection, in which only a partial-thickness band of sclera is removed. With the surgical closure of the wound, scleral buckling is achieved by the intrusion of the partially thinned sclera and choroid.

Custodis' segmental scleral buckle was extended and amplified by the development of an encircling scleral buckle by Schepens in 1953. He accomplished this by using a polyethylene tube that encircled the eye. However, the somewhat rigid encirclement led to the late complication of erosion of the sclera, choroid, and retina in some eyes. Therefore, polyethylene was replaced with silicone rubber, a softer polymer.

All of the early attempts to create an adhesive choroiditis employed an external approach. Then, in 1956, Meyer-Schwickerath introduced photocoagulation, with which chorioretinal lesions can be produced by a transpupillary route. This valuable method is now widely used for the treatment of retinal breaks without detachment and is occasionally applied postoperatively for additional treatment.

Although Bietti reported the use of cryosurgery for retinal detachment in 1933, it was Lincoff who developed this valuable method in 1964, and his reports on cryopexy have resulted in its widespread use. The major advantage of this freezing technique is the minimal damage to conjunctiva, muscle, and sclera. Transconjunctival treatment is therefore feasible, and the dissection of scleral flaps is not necessary.

A surgical approach to the vitreous, an important adjunct in selected cases, was pioneered by Shafer in 1950 with his method of vitreous transplantation. This important branch of surgery was expanded by Cibis in 1962 with his introduction of intravitreal silicone oil injection. The development of the vitreous infusion suction cutter (VISC) by Machemer in 1971 and the use of intravitreal sulfur hexafluoride gas by Norton in 1973 further expanded the role of vitreous surgery in the management of retinal detachment.

It is anticipated that the major area of future development in retinal reattachment will be the refinement of microscopic endosurgical techniques for the posterior segment, together with pharmacologic management of pathologic proliferations.

SUGGESTED READINGS

Arruga H: Gonin. *Am J Ophthalmol* 1965;60:659–662.

Custodis E: Scleral buckling without excision and with polyviol implant. In: Schepens CL, ed: *Importance of Vitreous Body with Special Emphasis on Reoperations.* St Louis: CV Mosby Co; 1960:175–182.

Gonin J: Treatment of detached retina by searing the retinal tears. *Arch Ophthalmol* 1930;4:621–625.

Jacklin HN: 125 years of indirect ophthalmoscopy. *Ann Ophthalmol* 1979;11:643–646.

Lincoff HA, McLean JM, Nano H: Cryosurgical treatment of retinal detachment. *Trans Am Acad Ophthalmol Otolaryngol* 1964;68:412–432.

Norton EWD: Intraocular gas in the management of selected retinal detachments. XXIX Edward Jackson Memorial Lecture. *Trans Am Acad Ophthalmol Otolaryngol* 1973;77:OP85–98.

Norton EWD: The past 25 years of retinal surgery. *Am J Ophthalmol* 1975;80:450–459.

CHAPTER 2

Pathogenesis and Natural History

Retinal detachment does not result from a single, specific disease; rather, it is the end result of numerous disease processes in which subretinal fluid is present. These include congenital malformations, metabolic disorders, traumatic changes, and vascular diseases.

2-1

TYPES OF RETINAL DETACHMENTS

The three types of retinal detachments are rhegmatogenous, exudative, and tractional. Both exudative and tractional detachments are sometimes referred to as *secondary* or *nonrhegmatogenous* detachments.

The three types of retinal detachments are not mutually exclusive. For example, cases of malignant melanoma have been seen in which the associated retinal detachment had a retinal break. A more common example is proliferative vitreoretinopathy, which exhibits both rhegmatogenous and tractional features. However, excluding the section on differential diagnosis (in Chapter 3), the scope of this monograph is limited to rhegmatogenous retinal detachments. Accordingly, throughout the monograph, the term *retinal detachment* refers to the rhegmatogenous type, unless another type is specifically mentioned.

2-1-1 Rhegmatogenous Detachments

Rhegmatogenous detachments (from the Greek *rhegma*, meaning a rent or fissure) are the most common. They are caused by a break in the retina through which fluid passes from the vitreous cavity into the subretinal space. Rhegmatogenous detachments are sometimes referred to as *primary* or *idiopathic* detachments. The break can be identified preoperatively in more than 90% of cases, but occasionally the presence of a minute, unseen break must be assumed.

2-1-2 Exudative Detachments

Exudative, or serous, detachments are due to an associated process, such as a tumor or an inflammation, that has produced subretinal fluid without a retinal break.

2-1-3 Tractional Detachments

Tractional detachments occur when pathologic vitreoretinal adhesions mechanically pull the retina away from the pigment epithelium. The most common causes include proliferative diabetic retinopathy, cicatricial retrolental fibroplasia, proliferative sickle retinopathy, and penetrating trauma.

2-2

EPIDEMIOLOGY OF RETINAL BREAKS

Several studies of eye bank eyes and nonselected clinical patients' eyes have revealed a 5% to 7% prevalence of retinal breaks in the general population. Most of these breaks are small atrophic holes near the ora that carry a low risk of subsequent retinal detachment. Equatorial horseshoe tears, which are associated with higher risk, are much less common.

2-3

EPIDEMIOLOGY OF RETINAL DETACHMENTS

Reliable information regarding the incidence and prevalence of retinal detachment is difficult to find because of the mobility of today's population. Several epidemiologic studies of relatively confined groups reveal an annual incidence of about 1 retinal detachment in 10,000. Assuming an average life expectancy of 74 years, the prevalence is approximately 0.7%.

The prevalence is considerably higher in certain groups. For instance, among people with high myopia, it is 5%. Among aphakic individuals, it is 2%; but if vitreous is lost at cataract extraction, the prevalence of detachment rises to 10%. The last figure has probably been reduced in recent years by improved surgical management of vitreous loss.

In one series of 104 asymptomatic patients with lattice degeneration, a 5-year followup disclosed that 0.2% had retinal detachment. If such a study were continued for 50 years, a prevalence of 2% could be expected.

2-3-1 Age

The most common age for retinal detachment is between 40 and 80 years, but a small group of patients have a peak incidence in their teens (Figure 2-1). In rare instances, detachment is discovered in a newborn, and occasionally it occurs as late as the ninth or tenth decade of life.

2-3-2 Sex

Approximately 60% of detachments occur in males. The incidence remains higher for males even when data are corrected for ocular trauma, which is more common among males than females. Except for high myopia (greater than 6 diopters), there are more male than female myopic patients in the general population, and the correlation between myopia and retinal detachments is well known.

2-3-3 Race

The incidence of detachment is reported to be relatively high among Jews and relatively low among African Americans. One study of Native Americans revealed an incidence essentially equal to that of the general Caucasian population.

2-3-4 Heredity

Primarily because myopia and lattice degeneration have hereditary tendencies, retinal detachment also has some hereditary predisposition. A positive family history of retinal detachment is a relevant risk factor, but most cases are sporadic.

2-3-5 Etiology

The most common associated features in retinal detachment are myopia, aphakia (including pseudophakia), lattice degeneration, and trauma. Approximately 40% to 55% of all detachment patients have myopia, 20% to 30% have lattice degeneration, and 10% to 20% have suffered direct ocular trauma. Approximately 30% to 40% of detachments are associated with surgical aphakia or pseudophakia, and the inci-

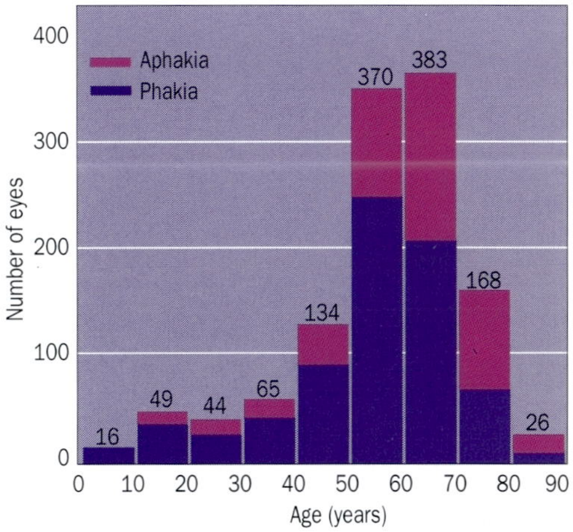

Figure 2-1 *Age distribution of retinal detachment patients with small juvenile mode and prominent middle-age mode.*

Redrawn with permission of S. Karger AG, Basel, from Hilton GF, Norton EWD: Juvenile retinal detachment. Mod Probl Ophthalmol *1969;8: 325–341.*

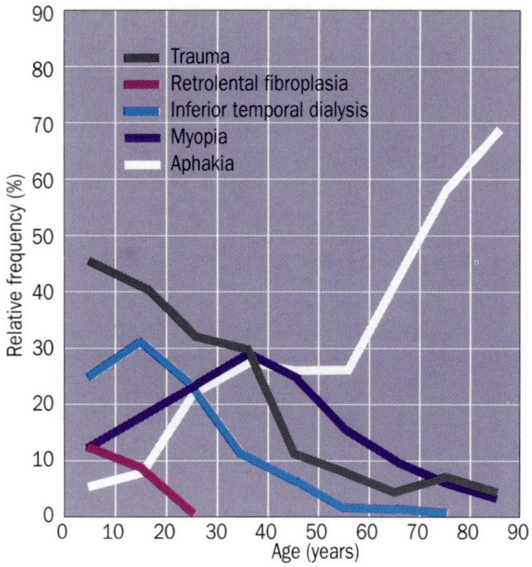

Figure 2-2 *Age distribution of five types of retinal detachment.*

Redrawn with permission of S. Karger AG, Basel, from Hilton GF, Norton EWD: Juvenile retinal detachment. Mod Probl Ophthalmol *1969;8: 325–341.*

dence increases when the posterior capsule is ruptured, when there is vitreous loss, or after YAG laser capsulotomy. Traumatic detachments are most common in youth, myopic detachments occur most frequently among people 25 to 45 years old, and the incidence of aphakic detachments rises with each decade of advancing age (Figure 2-2).

2-3-6 Bilaterality

Approximately 15% of detachment patients ultimately develop detachment in the second eye. The effect on bilaterality of prophylactic treatment, such as cryopexy of retinal breaks in the second eye at the time of detachment in the first eye, has not been evaluated. Bilateral detachments are more common in aphakic patients, with the incidence varying from 25% to 30%.

2-4

CLASSIFICATION OF RETINAL DETACHMENTS

Retinal detachments may be classified according to morphologic findings (Table 2-1).

2-5

RETINAL BREAKS

For rhegmatogenous retinal detachment to occur, there must be one or more retinal breaks, and liquid vitreous must have access to the break to get into the subretinal space. Posterior vitreous detachment, which usually precedes retinal detach-

TABLE 2-1

Classification of Detachments

Morphology of Break

- Horseshoe
- Round or oval
  - Operculated
  - Atrophic
- Dialysis
- Irregular

Etiology of Break

- Tractional
  - Horseshoe
  - Operculated
- Atrophic
- Postnecrotic

Location of Break

- Near ora serrata
- Equatorial zone
- Posterior to equatorial zone
- Macular

Number of Breaks

- Single
- Multiple

Size of Break

- Small
- Moderate
- Giant

Extent of Detachment

- One quadrant or less
- Two quadrants
- Three quadrants
- Four quadrants
- Total
- Detachment of pars plana epithelium

Secondary Changes

- Demarcation lines
  - Pigmented
  - Nonpigmented
- Intraretinal macrocysts
- Linear and angular strands on outer surface of detached retina (subretinal fibrosis)
- Microcystic degeneration of retina
- Thinning of retina
- Macular edema
- Macular hole
- Proliferative vitreoretinopathy (PVR)

ment, may lead to traction on the retina. Traction can cause breaks and may result in liquid vitreous being accessible to the break.

2-5-1 Types of Breaks

Retinal breaks may be subdivided into tears, holes, and dialyses (Table 2-2). Tears are produced by traction on the retina, whereas holes are due to gradual thinning of the retina. Tears occur suddenly, with the retina possibly appearing completely normal before the acute event.

TABLE 2-2

Types of Retinal Breaks

Type	Cause	Shape
Tear		
Horseshoe	Tractional	Flap
Operculated	Tractional	Round
Hole	Degenerative	Round
Dialysis	Traumatic or familial	Linear

Holes generally result from many years of antecedent retinal disease, and may be found within a patch of lattice degeneration, in retinoschisis, or in the thinned equatorial retina of the high myope.

Holes are generally round. Tears are often horseshoe-shaped and are called *horseshoe tears* or *flap tears*. However, tears can also be round when the portion of the retina where the vitreous is adherent pulls completely free from the surrounding retina. Called *operculated tears*, they can be distinguished from holes by the presence of the operculum, a small floater in the overlying vitreous representing the avulsed retina.

A retinal dialysis is a linear break of the retina, adjacent and parallel to the ora serrata. Dialyses are often caused by trauma. Familial and other nontraumatic retinal dialyses are also recognized.

2-5-2 Primary and Secondary Breaks

Retinal breaks are termed *primary* when they are responsible for production of the detachment. They are termed *secondary* when they are present preoperatively but are not responsible for the detachment and are subsequently lifted up by subretinal fluid. Secondary breaks also include those that develop in the retina after it detaches. There have been a few rare cases of secondary breaks appearing at the edge of paving-stone degeneration. Secondary breaks have also been seen at the site of old chorioretinal scars resulting from either inflammation or photocoagulation. A secondary break can also occur at the time of photocoagulation if excessive power is used. All breaks, both primary and secondary, should be treated at the time of surgery.

2-5-3 Incidence of Breaks

Several studies have shown a 5% to 7% incidence of retinal breaks in asymptomatic patients. Most are small atrophic retinal holes in the far periphery near the ora serrata. These holes are frequently covered by the vitreous base and only rarely lead to retinal detachment. Retinal flap tears appear most often in the equatorial zone, whereas retinal breaks with free opercula tend to be located more posteriorly. Because of the associated vitreous attachment, flap tears frequently lead to detachment, whereas a break with a free operculum will infrequently do so, lacking vitreous traction at the margin of the break. Retinal tears, with either attached flaps or free opercula, are most common in middle age, whereas retinal dialyses are most common in youth (Figure 2-3).

2-5-4 Vitreous Adhesions

The vitreous has a key role in the creation of retinal tears and subsequent detachment. In the normal adult eye, the vitreous adheres firmly to the retina at the vitreoretinal symphysis, or vitreous base. The zone of firm attachment is only 3 or 4 mm wide and straddles the ora serrata. A less firm adhesion of cortical vitreous to the retina is located around the optic disc and surrounding the macula. Occasionally, a tongue of vitreoretinal adhesion extends posteriorly from the vitreous base as far as the equator. Many areas of vitreoretinal attachment and traction are also found along retinal vessels and are accordingly termed *vitreovascular attachments*. This accounts for the frequent clinical presentation of a retinal tear as a vitreous hemorrhage and supports the clinical dictum that "a vitreous hemorrhage implies a retinal tear until proven otherwise." Pathologic adhesions frequently appear at the margin of a patch of lattice degeneration or at the site of previous chorioretinal inflammation.

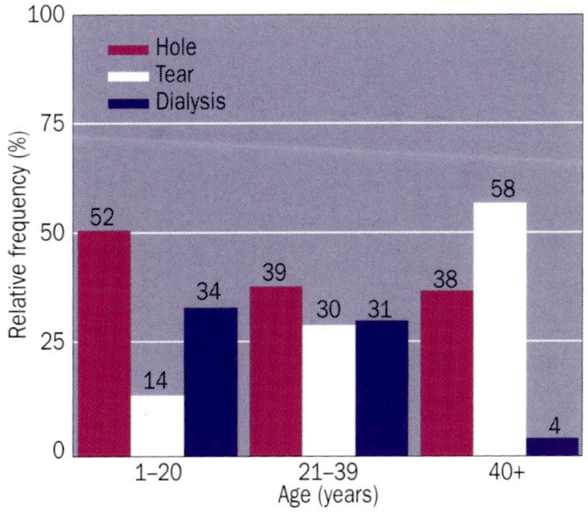

Figure 2-3 *Relative frequency of retinal breaks. Redrawn with permission of S. Karger AG, Basel, from Hilton GF, Norton EWD: Juvenile retinal detachment.* Mod Probl Ophthalmol *1969;8: 325–341.*

2-5-5 Horseshoe Tears

Also referred to as *flap*, *U-shaped*, or *arrowhead* tears, horseshoe tears occur in most cases at the irregular posterior margin of the vitreous base during posterior vitreous detachment. The flap thus remains adherent to the posterior vitreous surface following creation of a tear (Figure 2-4). Essential conditions for the produc-

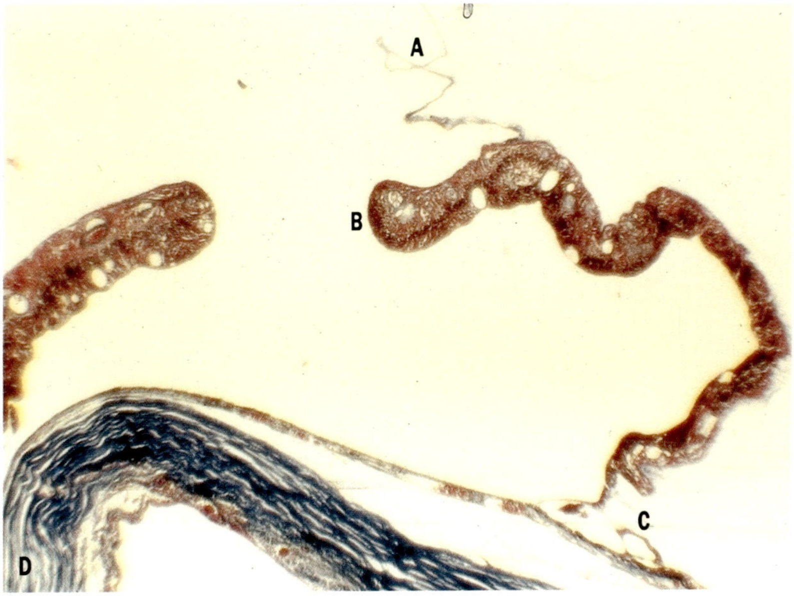

Figure 2-4 *Photomicrograph of horseshoe tear of retina with vitreous adherent to flap. (A) Vitreous. (B) Anterior edge of tear. (C) Ora serrata. (D) Sclera.*

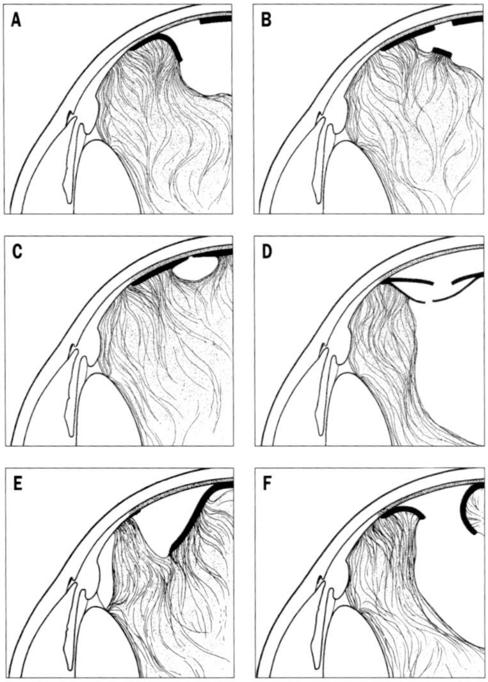

Figure 2-5 *Vitreoretinal relationships associated with retinal breaks. (A) Horseshoe tear with flap adherent to posterior hyaloid surface. (B) Tear with free operculum adherent to posterior hyaloid surface. (C) Atrophic hole caused by lattice degeneration. (D) Retinoschisis with holes in inner and outer layers producing retinal detachment. (E) Retinal dialysis with vitreous adherent to posterior edge of break. (F) Retinal dialysis with vitreous adherent to anterior edge of break.*

tion of a horseshoe tear are a pre-existing vitreoretinal adhesion and traction applied to this focus via the vitreous (Figure 2-5A).

2-5-6 Round Breaks With Free Opercula

Breaks with free opercula are produced by a mechanism similar to the one involved in horseshoe tears. However, the flap has been torn free from the retina at the anterior edge of the flap, and therefore the operculum is separated from the retina and adheres to the posterior hyaloid membrane (Figures 2-5B, 2-6). The breaks are caused by isolated areas of vitreoretinal adhesion and are not contiguous to the vitreous base. Operculated retinal breaks tend to be more posterior than horseshoe tears, and occasionally an operculated break is found posterior to a horseshoe tear in the same meridian.

2-5-7 Atrophic Holes

Atrophic holes are due to gradual thinning of the retina, often in association with lattice degeneration (Figure 2-5C). These small holes occur in the middle of the lattice patch and are distinguished from the retinal tears that occur in full-thickness retina at the margin of the lattice patch. The holes are due to atrophy, but the tears are related to vitreoretinal adhesions, which are universally found at the margin of lattice patches.

Retinoschisis is frequently accompanied by atrophic holes. Inner-layer holes are generally small and difficult to see. Outer-layer holes, which are larger and therefore more easily seen, are much more significant in the pathogenesis of retinal detachment (Figure 2-5D).

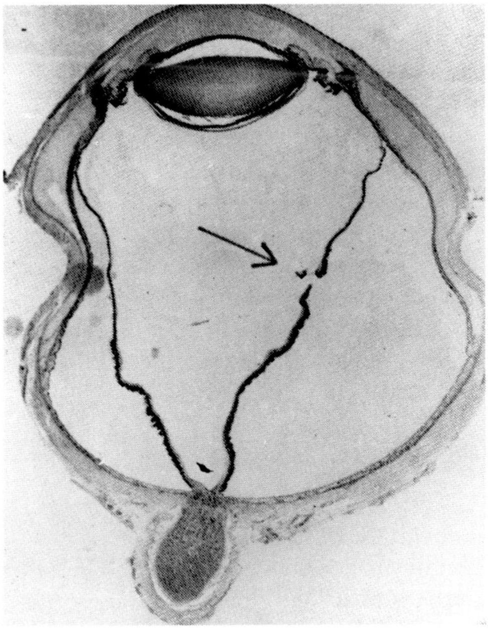

A

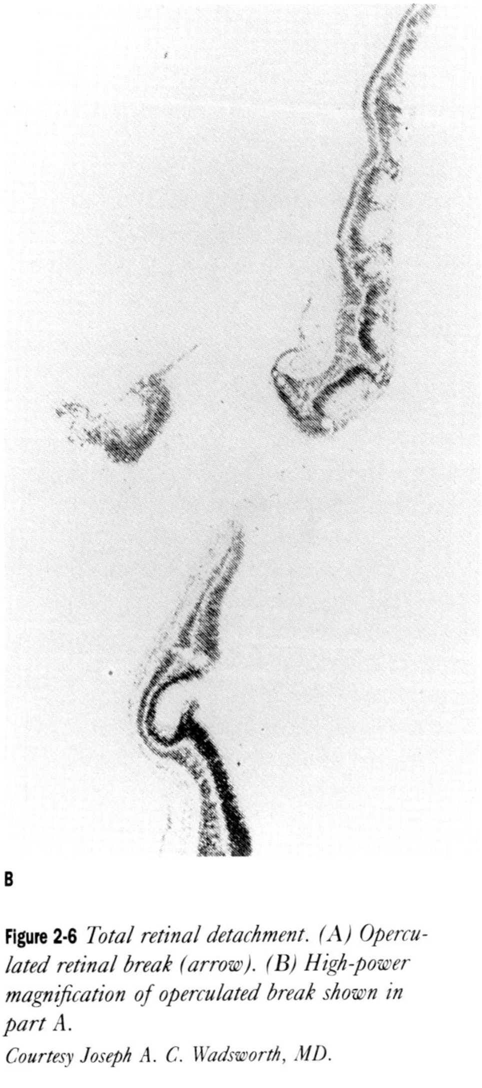

B

Figure 2-6 *Total retinal detachment. (A) Operculated retinal break (arrow). (B) High-power magnification of operculated break shown in part A.*

Courtesy Joseph A. C. Wadsworth, MD.

Atrophic holes sometimes occur in diffuse chorioretinal atrophy, such as in the equatorial zone of the highly myopic eye. In rare instances, they are caused by the rupture of a cystoid space in peripheral cystoid degeneration. However, in these cases, the holes seldom produce retinal detachments, because those at the extreme periphery are usually covered by the base of the vitreous.

2-5-8 Postnecrotic Holes

Postnecrotic holes can develop following retinitis. Cytomegalovirus (CMV) is a common cause of infectious retinitis in immunologically deficient patients such as patients on immunosuppressive therapy, fetuses in utero, and patients with acquired immune deficiency syndrome (AIDS). From 34% to 40% of patients with AIDS develop CMV retinitis, and of those who do, retinal detachment occurs in about 17%. These detachments typically are associated with multiple tiny postnecrotic holes.

Similar findings may be present with other forms of infectious retinitis, such as the acute retinal necrosis (ARN) syndrome. Postcontusional retinal necrosis with breaks also may develop following blunt trauma.

2-5-9 Macular Holes

Macular holes may be traction-induced or atrophic, operculated or nonoperculated. Gass has postulated that they often develop as a result of tangential traction from the vitreous cortex at the margins of the foveal pit. Macular holes may also be degenerative or may result from coalescence of intraretinal cystoid spaces. Trauma may also induce macular holes. The rare macular breaks that produce detachments are usually associated with trauma or high myopia.

2-5-10 Dialyses

A retinal dialysis is a circumferential linear tear, the anterior margin of which is at the ora serrata (Figure 2-5E). The retina is thinnest and least developed at the ora, especially in the inferior temporal quadrant. Dialyses occur at any age, but they are particularly common in youth—hence the well-known clinical entity of inferior temporal dialysis of the young. About 75% of retinal breaks that occur after blunt ocular trauma are retinal dialyses. Generally, the vitreous gel remains adherent to the posterior edge of torn retina. In this regard, dialyses are different from all other retinal tears in which the vitreous is attached to the anterior flap. A tear occurring quite anteriorly—for example, through an area of advanced peripheral cystoid degeneration related to the posterior edge of the vitreous base (Figure 2-5F)—might also be referred to clinically as a dialysis.

2-5-11 Traumatic Breaks

An uncommon type of dialysis is associated with circumferential tearing of a ribbon of the nonpigmented epithelium of the pars plana and the peripheral retina. The strip of epithelium and adherent vitreous tends to drape down as a festoon over the peripheral retina. This avulsion of the vitreous base is pathognomonic of antecedent ocular trauma (Figures 2-7, 2-8E). Traumatic dialysis can occur in any quadrant, but is said to be more common in the superior nasal quadrant. Pars plana breaks, which usually occur at the anterior limit of the vitreous base, are highly suggestive of trauma. In addition, macular holes and equatorial holes secondary to retinal necrosis constitute the major types of retinal breaks seen following contusion (see Figure 2-8).

2-5-12 Distribution of Breaks

The distribution of retinal breaks throughout the quadrants of the fundus is different for each type of break. Horseshoe tears are most common in the superior

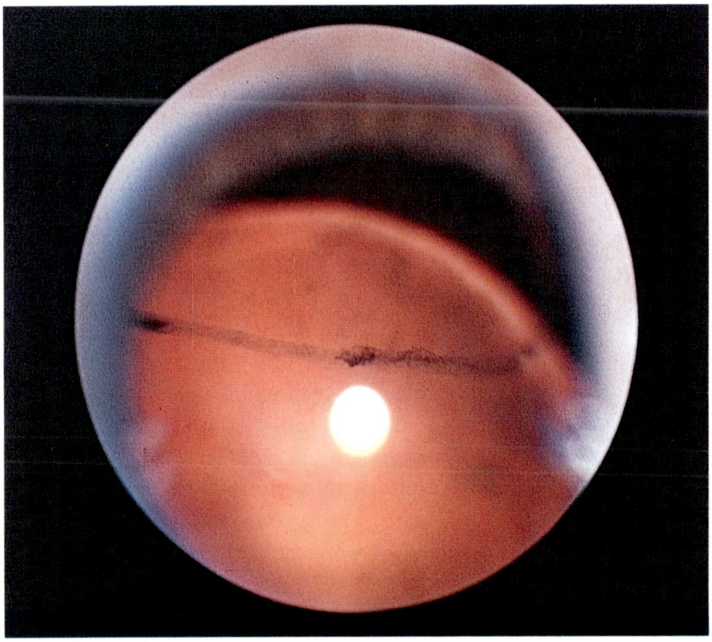

Figure 2-7 *Contused eye with avulsion of vitreous base and subluxated lens. Reproduced with permission of Medcom, Inc., from Conor O'Malley, MD, FACS, and Patrick O'Malley, MD, FACS: "The Peripheral Fundus of the Eye."*

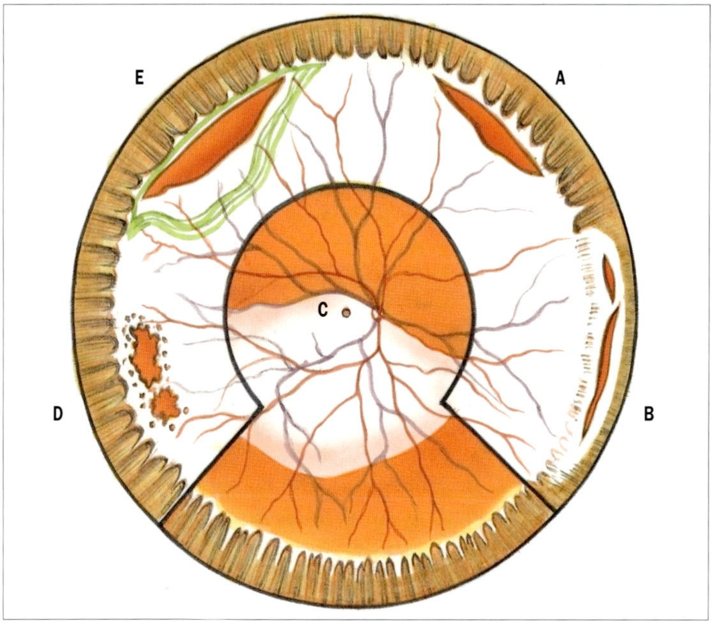

Figure 2-8 *Composite drawing showing five characteristic retinal breaks that may occur with ocular contusions. (A) Dialysis. (B) Pars plana breaks. (C) Macular break. (D) Postnecrosis break. (E) Avulsion of vitreous base (shown in green).*

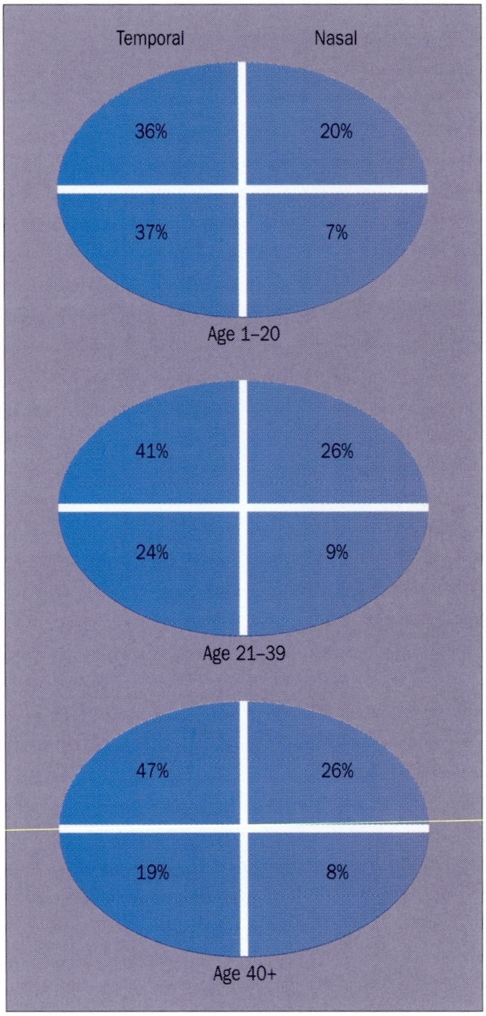

Figure 2-9 *Quadrantic distribution of retinal breaks by age group.*

Redrawn with permission of S. Karger AG, Basel, from Hilton GF, Norton EWD: Juvenile retinal detachment. Mod Probl Ophthalmol *1969;8: 325–341.*

temporal quadrant, and the second most susceptible site is the superior nasal quadrant. Therefore, tears tend to occur in the superior fundus. Atrophic retinal breaks are also usually located in the superior temporal quadrant, but the second most common quadrant is the inferior temporal. Thus, the principal site of atrophic breaks is the temporal fundus. Dialyses are found most frequently in the inferior temporal quadrant. The preponderance of superior temporal breaks in adults is not seen in juveniles because of the relatively high incidence of inferior temporal dialyses among youths (Figure 2-9).

In one large series of retinal breaks, 12% were found near the ora, 28% between the ora and the equator, 45% near the equator, 14% posterior to the equator, and 1% at the macula. In the typical aphakic detachment, one or more small retinal breaks are seen near the ora: equatorial breaks are relatively common in phakic eyes. In approximately 50% of retinal detachments, there is only one break. When there are multiple breaks, they are found to be within 90° of one another in 75% of the affected eyes.

2-6

LESIONS THAT CAUSE RETINAL BREAKS

Congenital anomalies and peripheral cystoid degeneration rarely lead to clinically significant retinal breaks. Although inner- or outer-layer breaks may develop in degenerative retinoschisis, it is the outer-layer breaks that will occasionally produce a clinical detachment of the retina. On the other hand, retinal breaks with lattice degeneration are common. Although the great majority of these breaks do not lead to retinal detachment, the condition is sufficiently common that 20% to 30% of retinal detachments are due to lattice.

2-6-1 Congenital Anomalies

Peripheral retinal variations can be sites of particular vitreoretinal adherence and traction at or just posterior to the vitreous base. Cystic retinal tufts (congenital retinal rosettes, granular patches, and glial spheres) and zonular traction tufts display such attachment, so that a retinal tear may be produced with or without posterior vitreous detachment.

2-6-2 Peripheral Cystoid Degeneration

Peripheral cystoid degeneration, occasionally seen in youth, is virtually universal in the far periphery of the senescent eye (Figure 2-10). Minimal cystoid degeneration is located immediately posterior to the ora serrata, and in more advanced cases it might extend as far posterior as the equator. This ubiquitous finding is generally insignificant, but in rare cases both the inner and the outer layers of a cyst rupture, creating a through-and-through retinal hole. The holes seldom lead to detachment because they are frequently covered by the vitreous base.

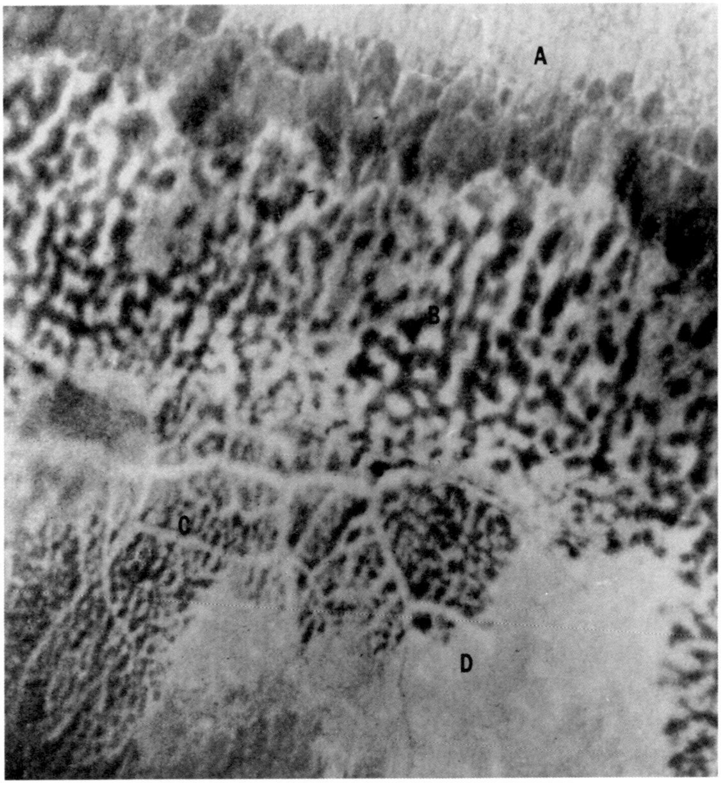

Figure 2-10 *Autopsy photograph of peripheral cystoid degeneration. (A) Pars plana. (B) Typical peripheral cystoid degeneration. (C) Reticular peripheral cystoid degeneration. (D) Normal retina.*

Reproduced from Straatsma BR, Foos RY: Typical and reticular degenerative retinoschisis. Am J Ophthalmol *1973;75:551–575. Published with permission from The American Journal of Ophthalmology. Copyright by The Ophthalmic Publishing Company.*

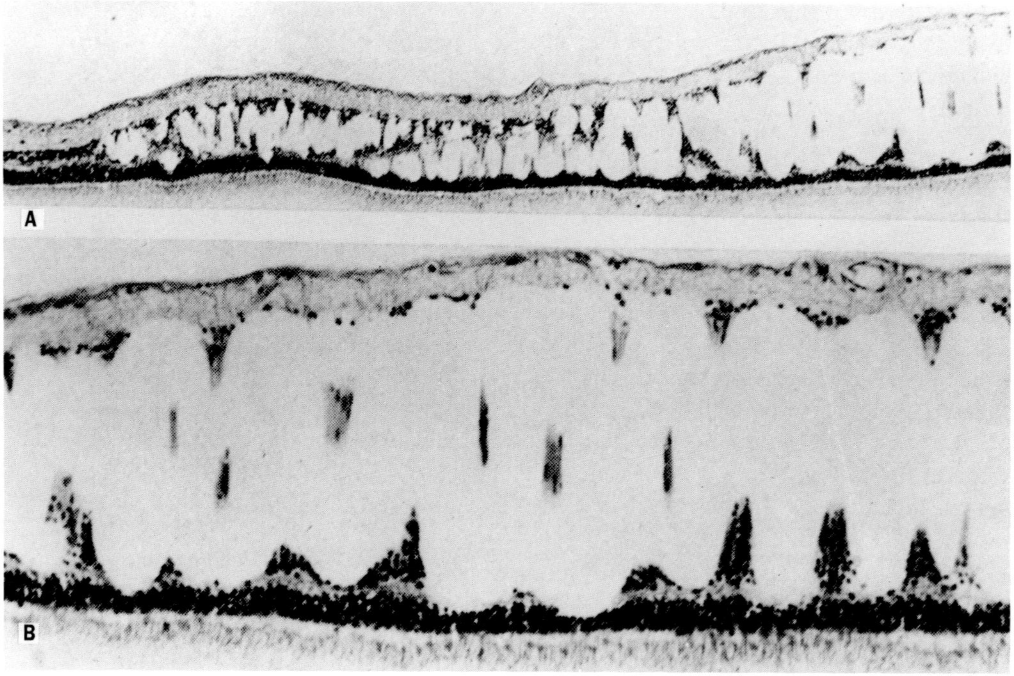

Figure 2-11 *Peripheral cystoid degeneration. (A) Photomicrograph. (B) Magnified view of part A.* *Reproduced from Straatsma BR, Foos RY: Typical and reticular degenerative retinoschisis.* Am J Ophthalmol *1973;75:551–575. Published with permission from The American Journal of Ophthalmology. Copyright by The Ophthalmic Publishing Company.*

The cystic process begins in the outer plexiform layer, but with enlargement can extend from the inner to the outer limiting membranes, with stretching of the Müller cell fibers that bridge the cystic space (Figure 2-11). When the stretched glial fibers give way, a frank splitting of the retina, referred to as *degenerative retinoschisis*, is produced.

2-6-3 Degenerative Retinoschisis

Degenerative retinoschisis results from the progression of peripheral cystoid degeneration and is usually bilateral. As the glial septa rupture and the small cysts coalesce, a splitting occurs (Figures 2-12, 2-13). There are two types: typical (flat) and reticular (bullous). Typical retinoschisis

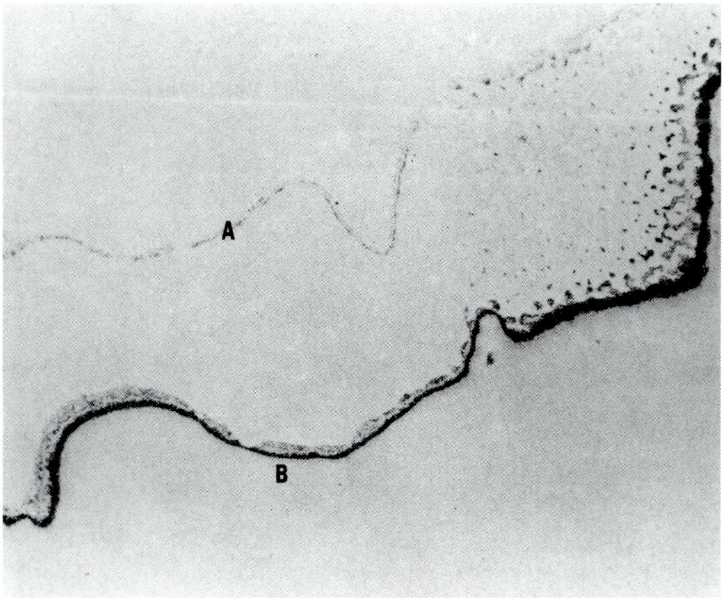

Figure 2-12 *Photomicrograph of retinoschisis, artifactually collapsed. (A) Inner layer. (B) Outer layer.* *Reproduced from Straatsma BR, Foos RY: Typical and reticular degenerative retinoschisis.* Am J Ophthalmol *1973;75:551–575. Published with permission from The American Journal of Ophthalmology. Copyright by The Ophthalmic Publishing Company.*

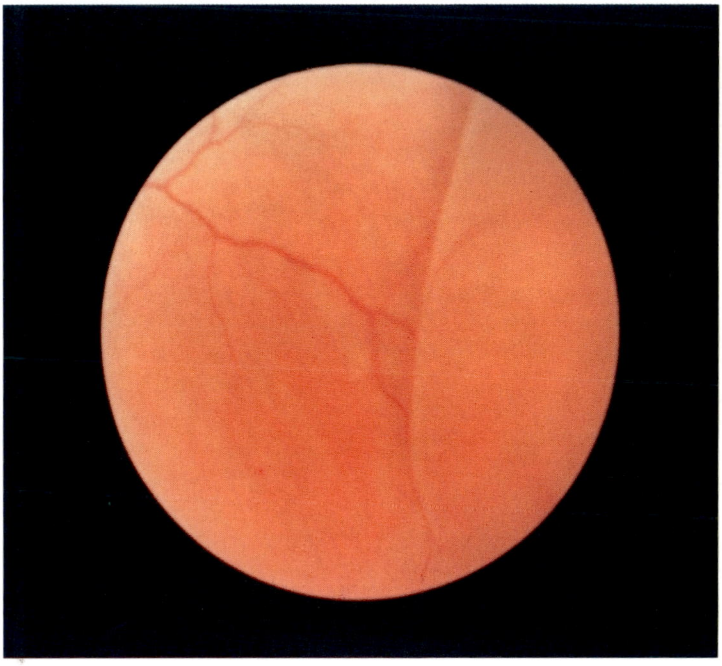

Figure 2-13 *Fundus photograph of retinoschisis.* *Reproduced with permission of Medcom, Inc., from Conor O'Malley, MD, FACS, and Patrick O'Malley, MD, FACS: "The Peripheral Fundus of the Eye."*

splits in the outer plexiform layer, is quite flat, and very rarely causes clinical retinal detachment. Reticular retinoschisis splits at the nerve fiber layer, is usually bullous, and is more likely to lead to clinical detachment.

Approximately 5% of the adult population has been found to have retinoschisis, generally of the flat type. The splitting may occur in any quadrant but is most common in the inferior temporal quadrant. Although splitting might extend posteriorly toward the macula, the most frequent avenue of extension is by circumferential progression around the periphery.

The inner layer of the bullous schisis cavity is extremely thin and characteristically exhibits multiple white flecks of uncertain etiology known as *snowflakes*. Blood vessels coursing over the dome of the retinoschisis frequently become sclerotic and are recognized by their white color. Inner-layer breaks are difficult to visualize with the ophthalmoscope. They tend to be multiple and are relatively small. The less common outer-layer break is more readily seen ophthalmoscopically, because it tends to range from 1 to 5 disc diameters in size and is often found posterior to the equator (Figure 2-14).

The outer layer usually remains adherent to the retinal pigment epithelium, and the rods and cones may be relatively well preserved though synaptically disconnected. As in peripheral cystoid degeneration, a mucopolysaccharide substance ex-

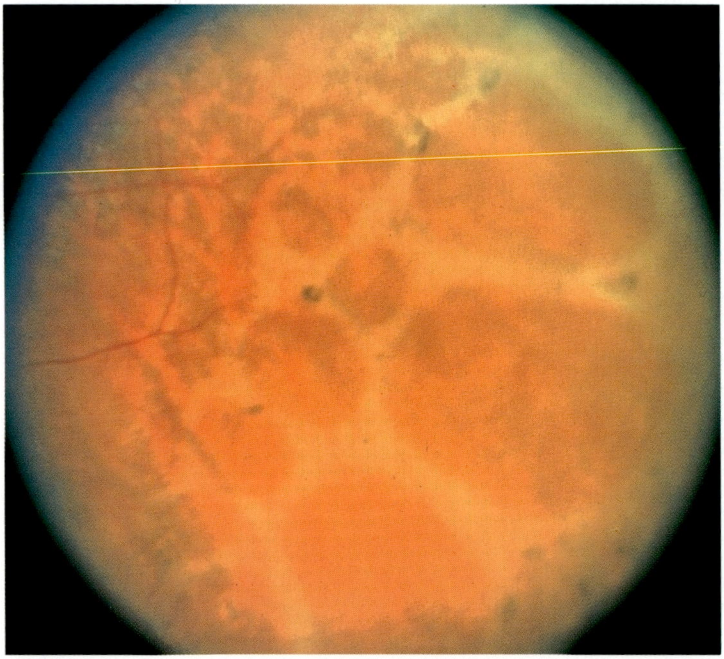

Figure 2-14 *Fundus photograph of retinoschisis with multiple outer-layer breaks.*
Courtesy C. P. Wilkinson, MD.

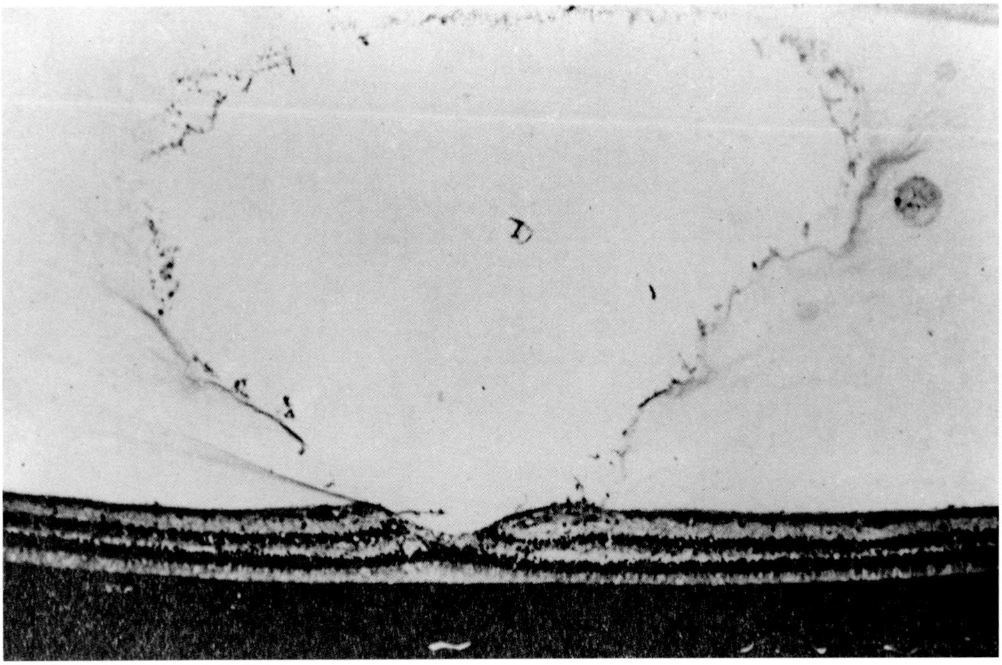

Figure 2-15 *Photomicrograph of lattice degeneration with prominent liquefaction of overlying vitreous cortex.*

ists within the schisis cavity that has been found to be sensitive to hyaluronidase. When retinoschisis produces retinal detachment, the subretinal fluid is derived from both the schisis and the vitreous cavities. The outer-layer breaks are usually visible, but there may be tiny inner-layer breaks that are not clinically detectable. It is the outer-layer breaks that are required for the development of detachment. Such detachments do not depend on the presence or absence of inner-layer breaks.

2-6-4 Lattice Degeneration

Lattice degeneration initially involves the vitreous cortex and the inner layers of the retina (Figure 2-15). As the lesion progresses, the outer layers also become in-

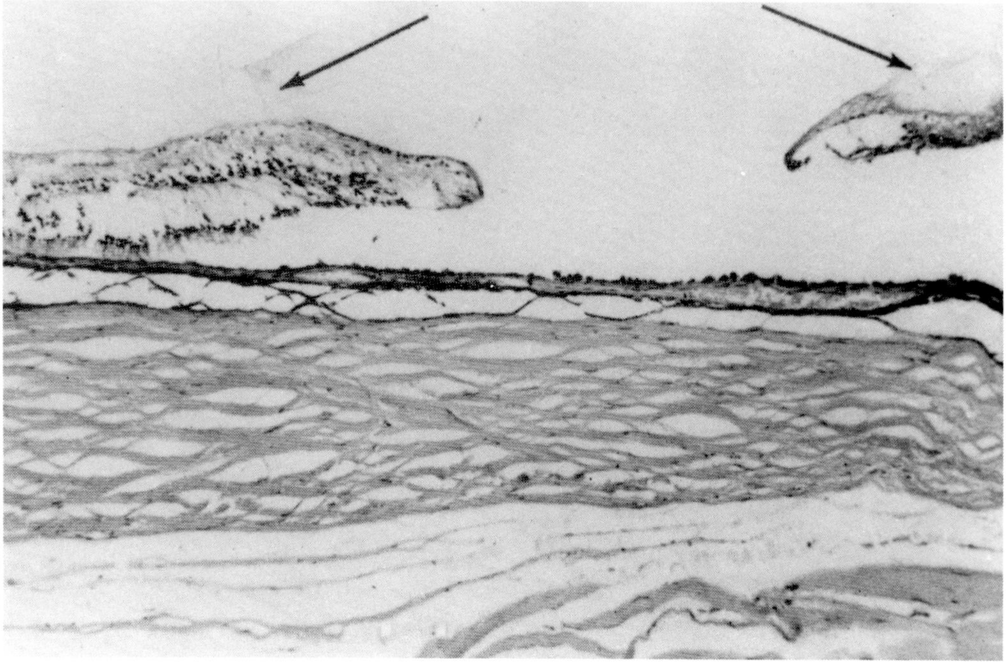

Figure 2-16 *Photomicrograph of lattice degeneration with atrophic hole, showing prominent vitreoretinal adhesions (arrows).*

Reproduced with permission from McPherson A, ed: New and Controversial Aspects of Retinal Detachment. *Philadelphia: Harper & Row; 1968.*

volved, and there may be sufficient thinning to cause through-and-through retinal holes (Figures 2-16, 2-17). The most consistent ophthalmoscopic feature of lattice degeneration is a circumscribed patch of excavation of the inner retinal surface. The patch is generally circumferential, oblong, and equatorial or pre-equatorial. Lattice degeneration varies in extent from a single isolated patch to almost continuous lesions around the equatorial zone of all four quadrants. There is usually just one plane of involvement between the ora and the equator, but occasionally there are two or three parallel rows, or tiers, of circumferentially oriented lattice. Infrequently, lattice is radial in its orientation, in which case it is generally in a perivascular distribution posterior to the equator.

Ophthalmoscopic examination reveals many variations in the appearance of lattice degeneration. In one form, referred to as *snail-track degeneration*, the lesion is completely white and almost reflective, with tiny, dot-like features on its surface. In most areas of lattice, the degenerative process is sufficiently deep to involve the pigment epithelium and there is derangement of pigment, with pigment clumping (Figure 2-18) and loss. In some lesions, there are fine, branching white lines due to sclerosis of the blood vessels passing through the lesion. (The term *lattice* is derived from this characteristic.) In general, fluorescein angiography of lattice lesions reveals a zone of relative avascularity. There may be small, round, atrophic holes due to retinal thinning in the patch of lattice and retinal tears at the edge of the patch (Figure 2-19) due to vitreoretinal adhesions. These tears are generally along

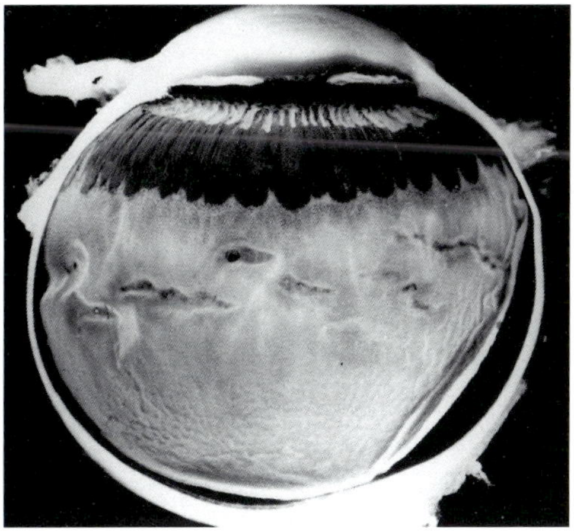

Figure 2-17 *Autopsy specimen with multiple patches of lattice degeneration.*

Reproduced with permission from Spencer LM, Straatsma BR, Foos RY: Tractional degenerations of the peripheral retina. In: Symposium on Retina and Retinal Surgery *(Transactions of the New Orleans Academy of Ophthalmology). St Louis: CV Mosby Co; 1969:103–127.*

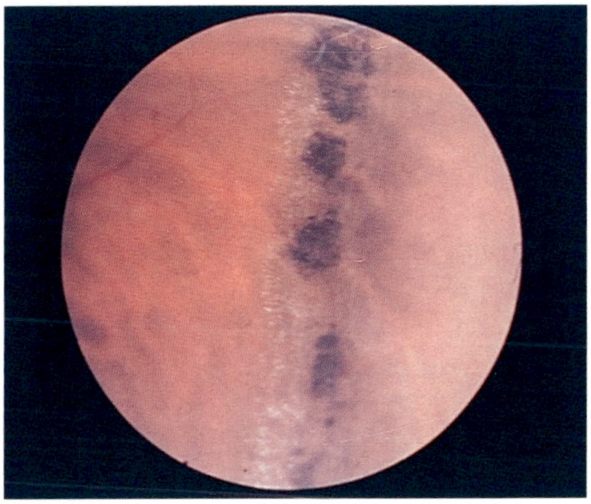

Figure 2-18 *Fundus photograph of lattice degeneration showing pigment clumps.*

Reproduced with permission of Medcom, Inc., from Conor O'Malley, MD, FACS, and Patrick O'Malley, MD, FACS: "The Peripheral Fundus of the Eye."

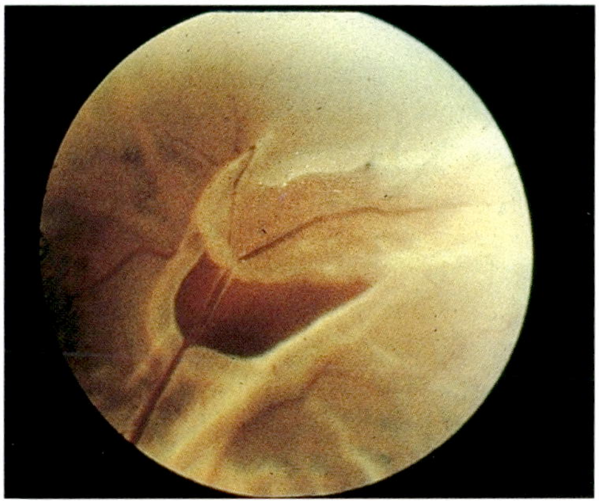

Figure 2-19 *Fundus photograph of lattice degeneration with horseshoe tear at one edge of lattice patch. Crossing the break is a "bridging vessel."*

the posterior edge of the lesion or at either end.

If posterior vitreous detachment is not present, only a small amount of fluid can pass through a lattice hole. This fluid is derived from the small pocket of vitreous liquefaction that overlies such lesions. A small amount of stable subretinal fluid, which is usually confined within the lattice patch, is therefore not regarded with the same concern as extensive subretinal fluid.

Lattice degeneration is found in all age groups, and new patches of lattice occur very rarely after the first decade of life. Changes within the lesion do occur, however, and many progressive features have been noted. Longitudinal observation has documented the subsequent appearance of pigmentation, branching white lines, retinal breaks, and subretinal fluid.

In one large series of 800 autopsy and 100 clinical eyes, lattice degeneration was found to be bilateral in 48% of cases, and more than one lesion was present in 50% of the 900 eyes examined. The lesions were parallel to the ora in 68% of the eyes, oblique in 25%, and perpendicular in 7%. Lesions that were close to the ora serrata were parallel to it, with the tendency for obliquity increasing progressively the more posterior the lesions were located. Lattice oriented perpendicular to the ora was usually quite posterior. Pigment clumping occurred in 92% of the lesions, retinal holes in 18%, white vessels in 7%, and retinal tears in 1.4%. Retinal tears were invariably accompanied by posterior vitreous detachment. It should be noted that the incidence of myopia in the series was higher than in the general population. As with myopia, there is a tendency for lattice to run in families.

2-6-5 Other Lesions

Rhegmatogenous detachments can also result from retinal breaks associated with Marfan syndrome, Ehlers-Danlos syndrome, Wagner's vitreoretinal degeneration/Stickler syndrome, Pierre-Robin syndrome, familial exudative vitreoretinopathy, juvenile retinoschisis, proliferative diabetic retinopathy, proliferative sickle retinopathy, retinopathy of prematurity, atopic dermatitis, acute retinal necrosis, and cytomegalovirus virus retinitis.

2-7

VITREOUS CHANGES PREDISPOSING TO DETACHMENT

A diagnosis of retinal detachment without posterior vitreous detachment, the most important vitreous change in the pathogenesis of retinal detachment, is rare (Figure 2-20). Posterior vitreous detachment is such a frequent phenomenon that it is regarded as a normal process of the aging eye. In one study, slit-lamp examination revealed that 65% of patients over age 65 had vitreous detachment. However, in a large series of autopsy eyes, only 22% had vitreous detachment by age 65, and 60% by age 75. In early life, the vitreous body is a homogenous gel consisting of a net-

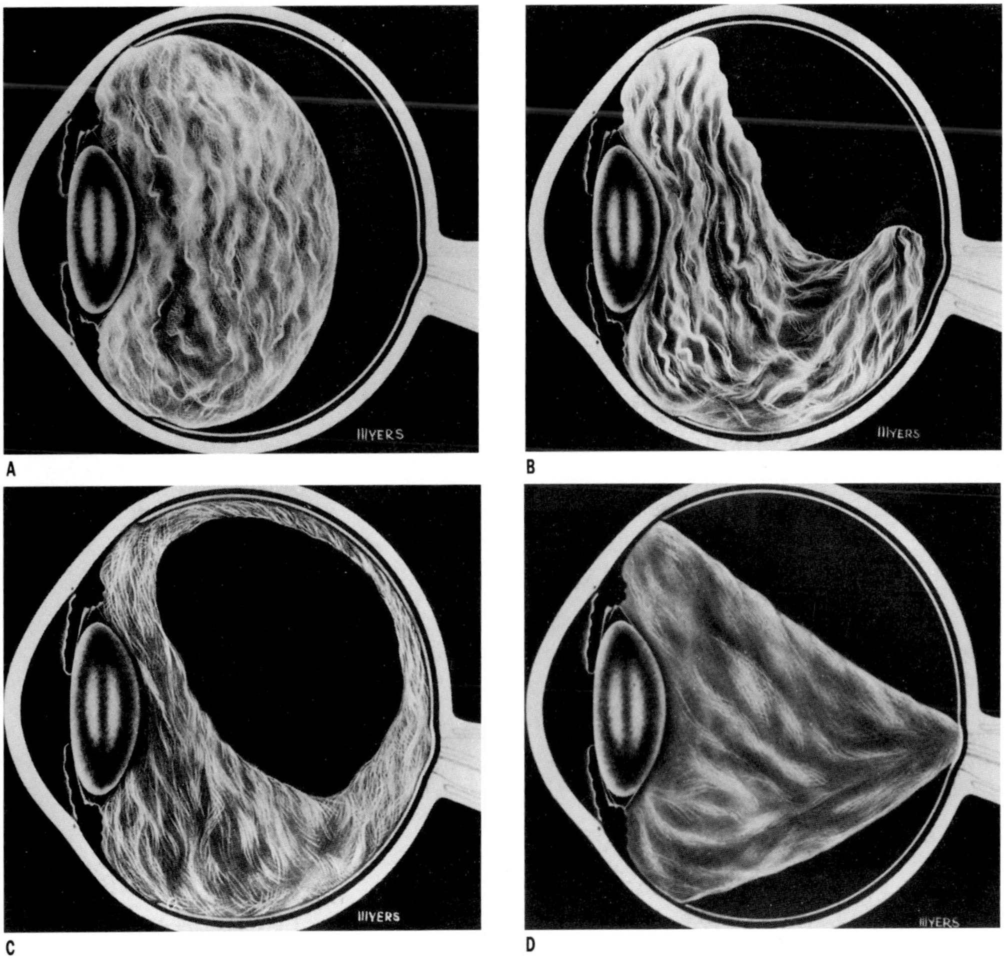

Figure 2-20 *Posterior vitreous detachment. (A) Complete and simple, without collapse. (B) With collapse. (C) Large posterior vitreous lacuna mimicking true posterior vitreous detachment. (D) Posterior vitreous detachment with persistent attachment at disc.*

Reproduced with permission from Jaffe NS: The Vitreous in Clinical Ophthalmology. *St Louis: CV Mosby Co; 1969.*

work of collagen fibrils separated from one another by macromolecules of hyaluronic acid. The density of fibrils is relatively higher near the retina and is highest at the vitreous base. The formed vitreous near the retina is referred to as the *vitreous cortex*.

With aging, the vitreous body undergoes loculation. Depolymerization and precipitation of the hyaluronic acid produces pockets of liquefaction or syneresis,

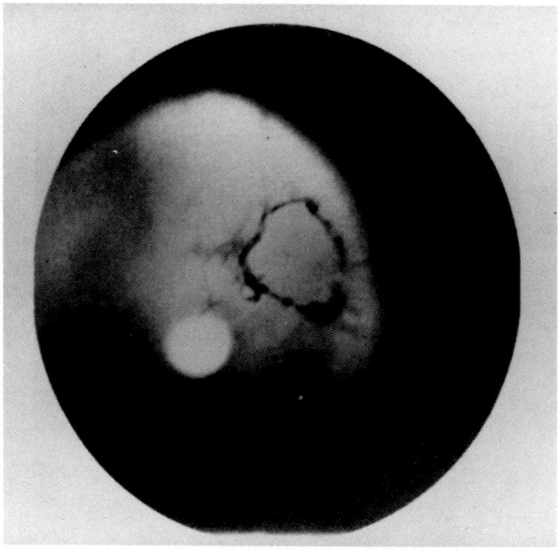

Figure 2-21 *Clinical photograph of midvitreal annular opacity (Weiss' ring), caused by posterior vitreous detachment pulling away from disc. Reproduced with permission from Jaffe NS: Macular retinopathy after separation of vitreoretinal adherence.* Arch Ophthalmol *1967;78:585–591. Copyright 1967 American Medical Association.*

which leads to lacunae formation. The thin collagen fibrils become matted and form prominent strands. This process, referred to as *fibrillar degeneration of the vitreous*, is often perceived by the patient as the onset of polymorphic floaters. The lacunae may coalesce, creating a large posterior cavity. Such a condition mimics posterior vitreous detachment in that a prominent vertical plane separating the anterior gel from posterior fluid vitreous can be seen on biomicroscopic examination. Detailed examination of the vitreous cortex is required to differentiate a large posterior lacuna from true posterior vitreous detachment. The former has been referred to as *pseudoposterior vitreous detachment.*

With rupture of the thin vitreous cortex, the intralacunar fluid enters the subhyaloid space and separates the vitreous body from the surface of the retina, producing true posterior vitreous detachment. The detachment generally starts posteriorly and proceeds peripherally toward the vitreous base. As the vitreous detaches from around the disc, it may pull loose a glial annulus, which the patient may see as a prominent floater (Weiss' ring) near the visual axis. The opacity is pathognomonic for posterior vitreous detachment (Figure 2-21). With collapse of the vitreous gel, the remaining formed vitreous assumes a position in the inferior aspect of the globe, a manifestation of the higher specific gravity of the gel. Because the vitreous remains firmly attached anteriorly, the pull of the collapsed gel frequently creates a fine circumferential retinal fold or ridge near the ora at the posterior limit of the vitreous base (Figure 2-22).

This sequence of events, normal to the aging eye, is often accelerated by contusion, cataract surgery, penetrating trauma with or without foreign bodies, diathermy, vitreous loss, inflammation, diabetes, or vitreous hemorrhage. Blood in the vitreous releases ferric ions from hemoglobin. These positively charged ions become fixed to negatively charged sites on hyaluronic acid, accelerating the depolymerization and precipitation of hyaluronic acid and resulting in collapse of the vitreous collagen structure.

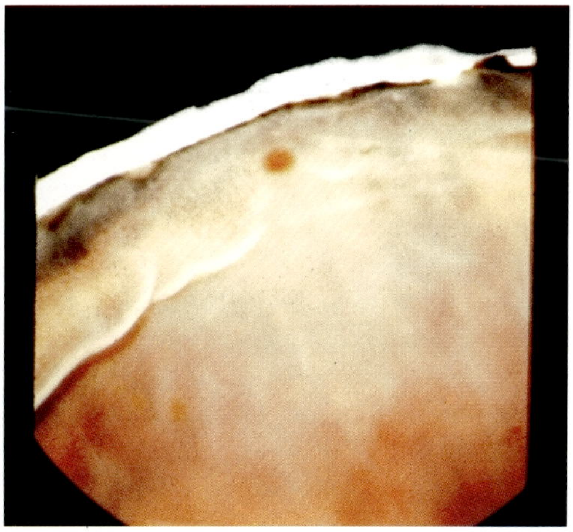

Figure 2-22 *Autopsy photograph of circumferential fold near ora caused by traction at posterior limit of vitreous base.*

2-7-1 Proliferative Diabetic Retinopathy

Vitreous changes are instrumental in the production of the retinal detachment in proliferative diabetic retinopathy. Numerous vitreoretinal adhesions form prior to separation of the posterior hyaloid. As the vitreous detaches, the retina may be focally elevated as a traction retinal detachment. Occasionally, a splitting phenomenon occurs, producing secondary retinoschisis, especially along retinal vessels. This process may produce retinal breaks. The typical rhegmatogenous detachment of proliferative diabetic retinopathy starts as a detachment of the posterior retina with small traction-related breaks, from which the retinal detachment subsequently spreads to the ora serrata.

2-7-2 Inflammation

Intraocular inflammatory changes may alter the vitreous and thereby predispose to retinal detachment through the production of vitreous traction bands or a transvitreal membrane, especially a cyclitic membrane.

2-7-3 Trauma

Trauma to the vitreous may induce changes that lead to retinal detachment many months after the initial injury. The classic retinal break in contusion is an anterior retinal dialysis. The dialysis is thought to result from the marked deformation of the globe, which, in association with the relatively inelastic vitreous base, tears the peripheral retina. The pathognomonic avulsion of the vitreous base has been mentioned previously. Penetrating trauma is often followed by the appearance of a dense vitreous band along the track of the injury, and the band may contract, which subsequently detaches the retina.

Surgical trauma may be responsible for, or contribute to, changes in the vitreous that increase the likelihood of retinal detachment. Besides accelerating posterior vitreous detachment via hyaluronic acid breakdown, cataract extraction can alter vitreous dynamics by displacement alone. Traction of varying degrees may develop along the vitreous base following uncomplicated surgery and certainly after vitreous loss.

Because the posterior capsule is left intact in the majority of modern cataract operations, posterior capsulotomy by Nd:YAG laser has become a frequent secondary procedure. Accelerated hyaluronic acid changes and vitreous degeneration increase the incidence of retinal tears and detachment after posterior capsulotomy.

2-8

PATHOGENESIS OF RETINAL DETACHMENT

If retinal breaks and posterior vitreous detachment are common, why does clinical detachment of the retina occur so infrequently? Whether or not fluid vitreous passes through a retinal break depends on the balance of forces operative at the edge of the break. Forces normally responsible for retinal attachment include negative pressure in the subretinal space created by the metabolic pump of the retinal pigment epithelium and the relatively higher oncotic pressure in the choroid, interdigitation of the pigment epithelial cell processes and the outer segment of photoreceptors, and mucopolysaccharide "glue" between the pigment epithelium and the sensory retina. Pigment epithelial hyperplasia around the break may create a small annular adhesion, which is recognized clinically as a demarcation line. Occasionally, some inflammatory cells producing a low-grade chorioretinitis are found around the break. Cortical vitreous may impede fluid movement across the retina or its access to retinal breaks.

In contrast, factors that tend to promote the passage of liquid vitreous through a break into the subretinal space include ocular movement, gravity, vitreous traction at the edge of the break, and posterior vitreous detachment, which allows access of subhyaloid fluid to the break.

The source of the subretinal fluid has been the subject of some controversy. The concentration of ascorbic acid is relatively high in the vitreous, and is higher in the subretinal fluid than in the plasma. This supports the concept that fluid vitreous passes through the retinal break into the subretinal space. With the passage of time, the concentration of ascorbic acid in the subretinal fluid decreases, which suggests that serum from the choriocapillaris has entered the subretinal space. The latter concept is supported by the observation that in a recent detachment the serum protein concentration in subretinal fluid is rather low but rises with time. A dual origin of subretinal fluid is most likely, with the major initial source being the liquid vitreous, which is subsequently augmented by serum from the choriocapillaris.

2-9

PATHOLOGY OF THE DETACHED RETINA

The outer layers of the detached retina undergo the greatest alteration due to separation from the blood supply of the choriocapillaris. Microcystoid spaces typically develop in the outer plexiform layer, although similar changes have been found in the middle and inner retinal layers. The changes can be reversed by surgical reattachment.

The inner and outer nuclear layers of the detached retina undergo degeneration, become thinner, and may ultimately fuse into one layer. Although the inner retina is well preserved initially, the ganglion cells decrease in number in long-standing detachments and may eventually disappear (Figure 2-23). Other chronic changes in-

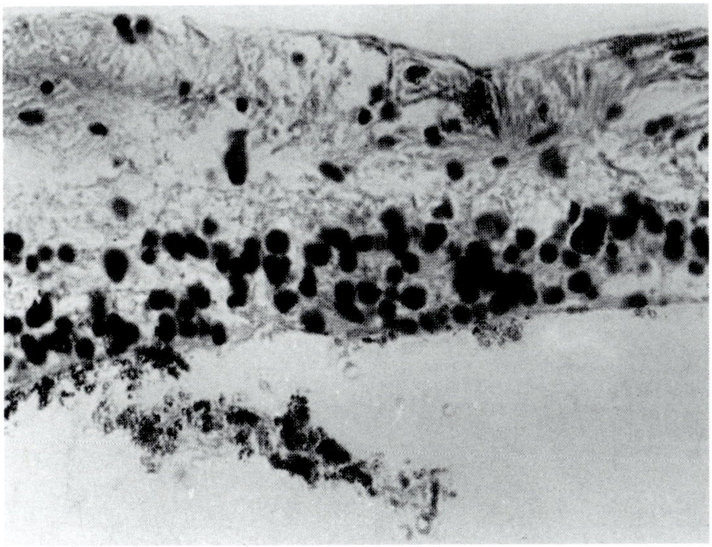

Figure 2-23 *Photomicrograph of long-standing retinal detachment showing loss of nuclear elements in retina, with complete absence of ganglion cells, some fragments of rods and cones, and dispersion of pigment epithelial cells.*

Courtesy Joseph A. C. Wadsworth, MD.

Figure 2-24 *Electron photomicrographs of photoreceptor outer segments in owl monkey. (A) Normal segments. Stacks of flattened membranous saccules (S) are enclosed by cytoplasmic membranes (C).*

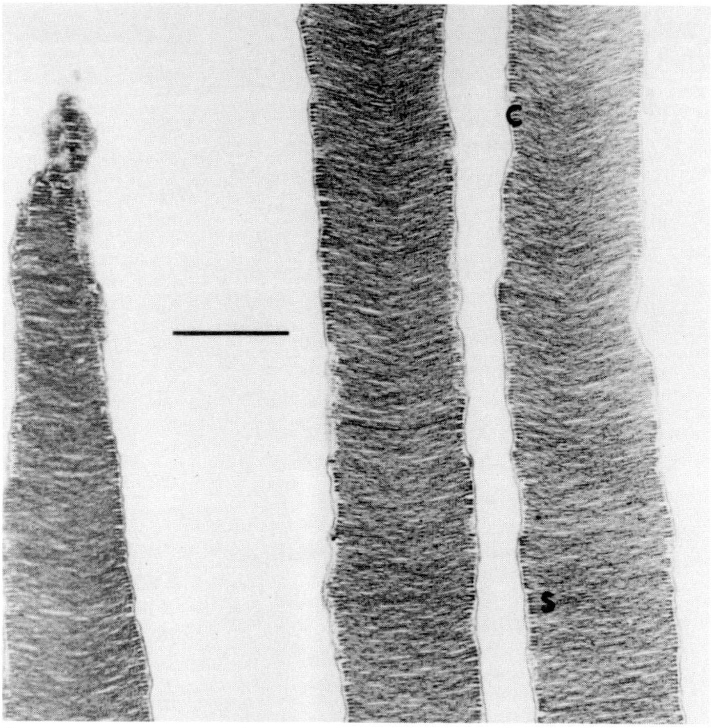

A

clude hyalinization of both retinal vessels and the choriocapillaris.

Experimental work with the owl monkey has revealed degenerative changes in the outer segments of the receptor cells within a few days after detachment (Figure 2-24). The discs of the outer segments become ruptured and disorganized and, in time, assume bizarre shapes. In the normal retina, shed fragments of photoreceptor outer segments are phagocytosed by the retinal pigment epithelium. These lamellar inclusion bodies are referred to as *phagosomes*. In retinal detachment, this process is disrupted so that phagosomes disappear from the retinal pigment epithelium. Both proliferative and degenerative changes occur in the retinal pigment epithelium. Changes visible with an electron microscope include migration of the pigment granules from the anterior processes of the retinal pigment epithelial cells posteriorly and thickening of Bruch's membrane. After surgical reattachment, the receptor cell outer segments regenerate, the

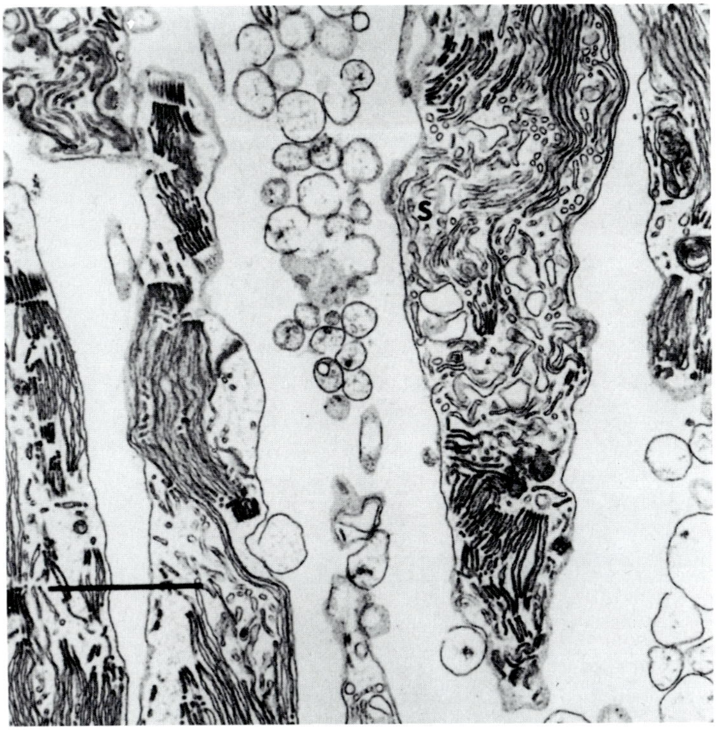

B

Figure 2-24 *(B) Degeneration of segments 1 week after retinal detachment. Saccules (S) are abnormally arranged and fragmented. Reproduced with permission from Kroll AJ, Machemer R: Experimental retinal detachment and reattachment, II: electron microscopy. In:* Symposium on Retina and Retinal Surgery *(Transactions of the New Orleans Academy of Ophthalmology). St Louis: CV Mosby Co; 1969: 258–277.*

discs assume a more normal pattern, and phagosomes reappear in the retinal pigment epithelial cells.

2-9-1 Intraretinal Macrocysts

Large intraretinal cystoid spaces may develop over many months in long-standing retinal detachments (Figures 2-25, 2-26). These macrocysts usually protrude into the subretinal space. They may develop in the posterior pole but are more frequent in the equatorial zone. Retinal detachments caused by inferior retinal breaks, such as the classic inferior temporal dialysis of the young, are generally

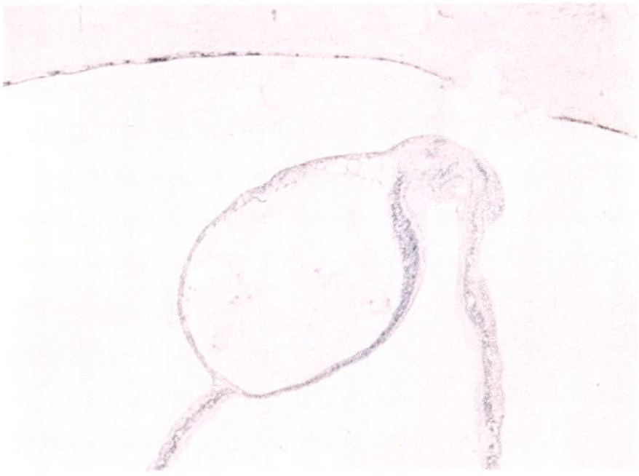

Figure 2-25 *Photomicrograph of intraretinal macrocyst.*

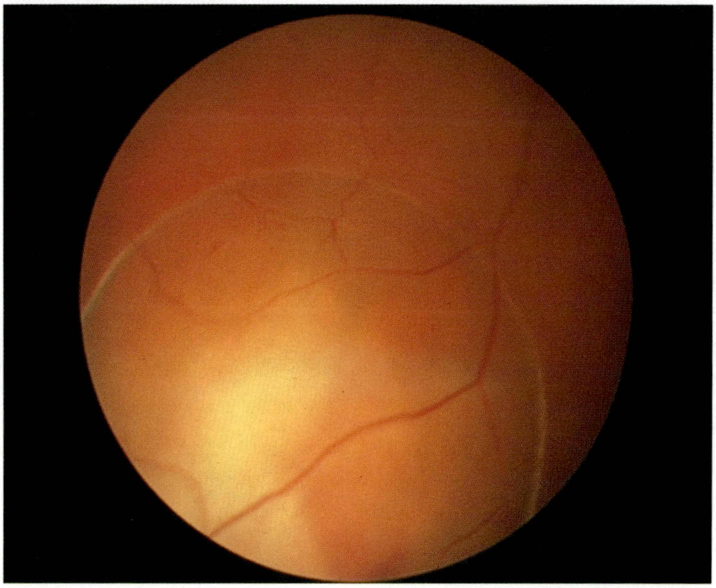

Figure 2-26 *Fundus photograph of intraretinal macrocyst.*
Courtesy Norman E. Byer, MD.

slow in their progression and thus may be present long enough to develop macrocysts before the detachment becomes symptomatic. Conversely, macrocysts are relatively rare in retinal detachments caused by superior breaks. With surgical reattachment, the macrocysts regress rapidly.

2-9-2 Demarcation Lines

If the boundary of a retinal detachment remains stable for a long time, pigment epithelial hyperplasia occurs at the junction between detached and attached retina. It is generally accepted that a minimum of 3 months is required to generate a demarcation line (also referred to as *friction line* or *high-water mark*). The to-and-fro undulations of the retina probably have an irritating effect on the retinal pigment epithelium at the boundary and induce a proliferative change, which subsequently evolves to fibrous metaplasia (Figure 2-27). Most demarcation lines have prominent pigmentation, but occasionally the pigment granules are lost and nonpigmented demarcation lines result. In rare cases, calcification of the line occurs in long-standing detachments. Demarcation lines may create a permanent barrier to the further progression of the detachment, but often the detachment extends through

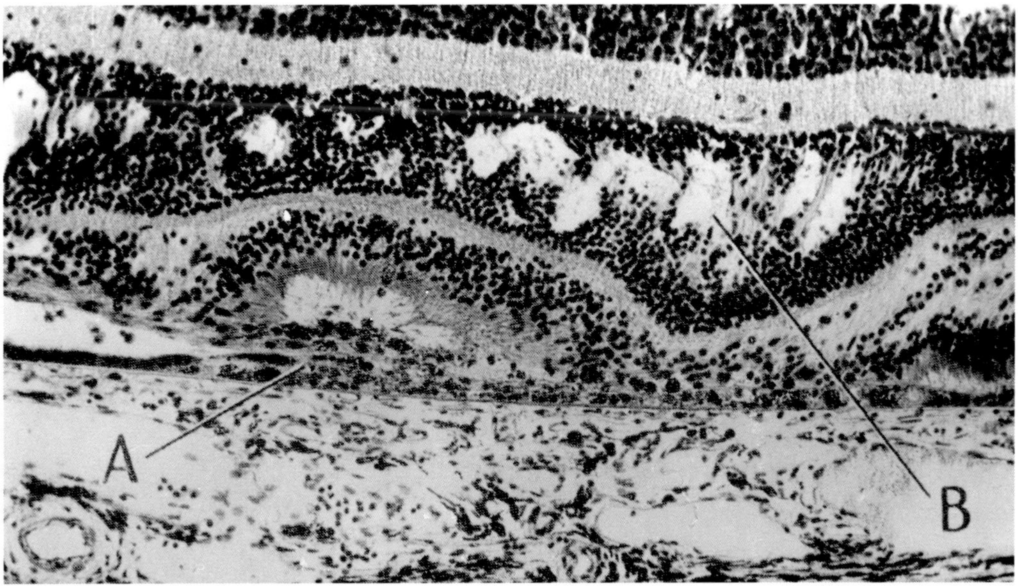

Figure 2-27 *Photomicrograph of demarcation line showing (A) fibrous metaplasia of retinal pigment epithelium and (B) microcystoid degeneration of outer nuclear layer.*

Courtesy Joseph A. C. Wadsworth, MD.

the barrier and progresses posteriorly. Several concentric demarcation lines may appear, indicating intermittent extension and temporary stability in the course of detachment.

2-9-3 Proliferative Vitreoretinopathy

The most ominous and clinically significant finding in retinal detachment is the presence of proliferative vitreoretinopathy (PVR). The consequence of cell migration and elaboration of collagen is the formation of membranes involving the inner and outer surfaces of the retina, as well as the vitreous. In time, and under the influence of mediators of inflammation, the membranes contract, distorting the retina into folds (Figure 2-28). Localized contracture

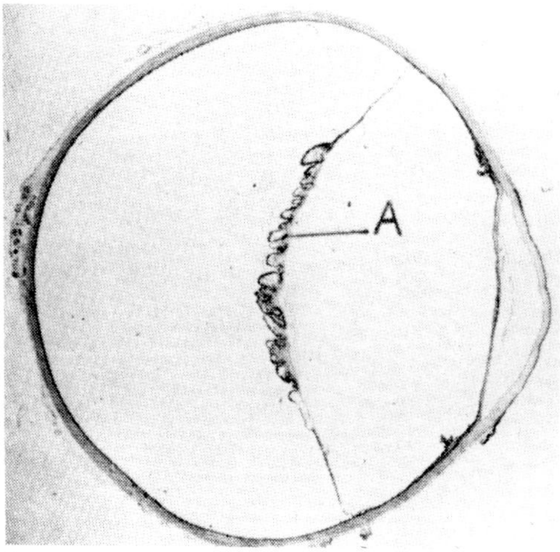

A

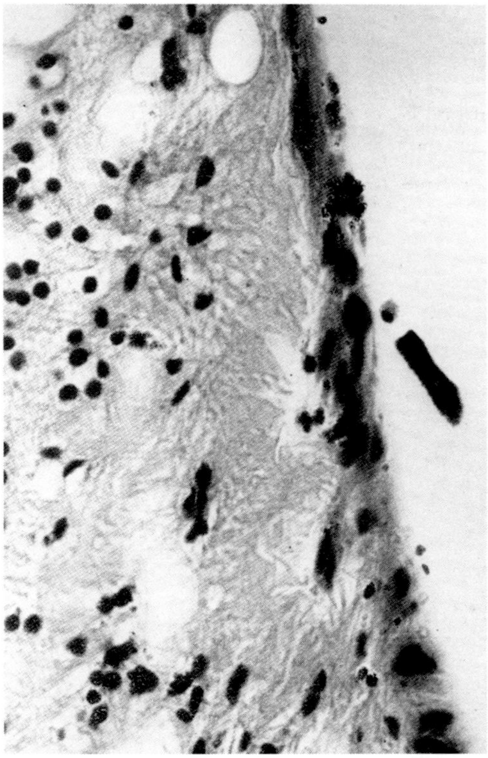

B

Figure 2-28 *Proliferative vitreoretinopathy. (A) Photomicrograph of total retinal detachment with marked corrugation of retina. (B) High-power magnification of part A, showing cellular preretinal membrane.*
Courtesy Joseph A. C. Wadsworth, MD.

in the periphery is referred to as a *star fold*, and a similar process in the posterior pole is referred to as a *macular pucker*. PVR, which used to be known as *massive vitreous retraction* (MVR) or *massive periretinal proliferation* (MPP), accounts for the majority of inoperable or unsuccessfully operated retinal detachments. Two recent classification systems for PVR have come into use and, though imperfect, they have improved our evaluation of retinal detachment and its therapy. (For further discussion of proliferative vitreoretinopathy, see Section 3-16.)

2-9-4 Subretinal Changes

Subretinal fluid usually contains sufficient protein to be stained as eosinophilic material to distinguish true from artifactitious detachment in the pathology laboratory. In long-standing detachments, the subretinal fluid may also contain macrophages, proliferating pigment cells, and cholesterol crystals from past hemorrhaging.

2-10

NATURAL HISTORY OF UNTREATED DETACHMENT

A limited retinal detachment may follow one of four outcomes:

1. Very rarely, spontaneous closure of the retinal hole by scar tissue leads to reattachment.

2. Infrequently, a detachment due to a superior retinal break settles inferiorly, and the site of the original break flattens.

3. Occasionally, a detachment remains indefinitely as a subtotal detachment with stable borders and the creation of demarcation lines. This is most apt to occur in detachments caused by inferior breaks.

4. Usually, most detachments progress to total detachment.

Late secondary changes include cataract and alterations of intraocular pressure. Occasionally, the low-grade uveitis that accompanies retinal detachment damages the trabecular meshwork enough to produce elevated intraocular pressure. The glaucoma of other long-standing detachments may be secondary to rubeosis iridis and is comparable to other forms of neovascular glaucoma. On the other hand, the uveitic process or traction on the ciliary body by proliferative vitreoretinopathy may decrease the production of aqueous humor to the point of hypotony and eventual phthisis.

Clinically, proliferative vitreoretinopathy is seen most often after surgery, but it is also observed as the end result of the natural history of unoperated retinal detachment.

SUGGESTED READINGS

Aaberg TM, Stevens TR: Snail track degeneration of the retina. *Am J Ophthalmol* 1972; 73:370–376.

Byer NE: Cystic retinal tufts and their relationship to retinal detachment. *Arch Ophthalmol* 1981;99:1788–1790.

Byer NE: Long-term natural history of lattice degeneration of the retina. *Ophthalmology* 1989;96:1396–1401.

Byer NE: Long-term natural history study of senile retinoschisis with implications for management. *Ophthalmology* 1986;93:1127–1137.

Byer NE: The natural history of asymptomatic retinal breaks. *Ophthalmology* 1982;89: 1033–1039.

Byer NE: *The Peripheral Retina in Profile: A Stereoscopic Atlas.* Torrance, CA: Criterion Press; 1982, slides 34, 119.

Celorio JM, Pruett RC: Prevalence of lattice degeneration and its relation to axial length in severe myopia. *Am J Ophthalmol* 1991;112: 356–357.

Combs JL, Welch RB: Retinal breaks without detachment: natural history, management and long-term follow-up. *Trans Am Ophthalmol Soc* 1982;80:64–97.

Cox MS, Freeman HM: Retinal detachment due to ocular penetration, I: clinical characteristics and surgical results. *Arch Ophthalmol* 1978;96:1354–1361.

Davis MD: Natural history of retinal breaks without detachment. *Arch Ophthalmol* 1974; 92:183–184.

Dumas J, Schepens CL: Chorioretinal lesions predisposing to retinal breaks. *Am J Ophthalmol* 1966;61:620–630.

Ebert EM, Mukai S: Familial exudative vitreoretinopathy. *Int Ophthalmol Clin* 1993;33: 237–247.

Flynn JT, Bancalari E, Bachynski BN, et al: Retinopathy of prematurity: diagnosis, severity, and natural history. *Ophthalmology* 1987; 94:620–629.

Foos RY: Posterior vitreous detachment. *Trans Am Acad Ophthalmol Otolaryngol* 1972;76: 480–497.

Foos RY: Tears of the peripheral retina: pathogenesis, incidence and classification in autopsy eyes. *Mod Probl Ophthalmol* 1975;15:68–81.

Freeman HM, Cox MS, Schepens CL: Traumatic retinal detachments. *Int Ophthalmol Clin* 1974;14:151–170.

Freilich DB, Seelenfreund MH: Miotic drugs, glaucoma, and retinal detachment. *Mod Probl Ophthalmol* 1975;15:318–322.

Goldberg MF: Retinal detachment associated with proliferative retinopathies. *Ophthalmic Surg* 1971;2:222–231.

Griffith RD, Ryan EA, Hilton GF: Primary retinal detachments without apparent breaks. *Am J Ophthalmol* 1976;81:420–427.

Grignolo A, Schepens CL, Heath P: Cysts of the pars plana ciliaris. *Arch Ophthalmol* 1957; 58:530–543.

Grizzard WS, Hilton GF: Scleral buckling for retinal detachments complicated by periretinal proliferation. *Arch Ophthalmol* 1982;100: 419–422.

Gutman FA, Zegarra H: Retinal detachment secondary to retinal branch vein occlusion. *Trans Am Acad Ophthalmol Otolaryngol* 1976; 81:491–496.

Hagler WS: Retinal dialysis as the cause of a special type of retinal detachment. *South Med J* 1965;58:1475–1482.

Hagler WS, North AW: Intraretinal macrocysts and retinal detachment. *Trans Am Acad Ophthalmol Otolaryngol* 1967;71:442–454.

Hagler WS, Woldoff HS: Retinal detachment in relation to senile retinoschisis. *Trans Am Acad Ophthalmol Otolaryngol* 1973;77:OP99–113.

Hirose T, Lee KY, Schepens CL: Snowflake degeneration in hereditary vitreoretinal degeneration. *Am J Ophthalmol* 1974;77:143–153.

Irvine AR: The pathogenesis of aphakic retinal detachment. *Ophthalmic Surg* 1985;16:101–107.

Kraushar MF, Steinberg JA: Miotics and retinal detachment: upgrading the community standard. *Surv Ophthalmol* 1991;35:311–316.

Kroll AJ, Machemer R: Experimental retinal detachment in the owl monkey, 8: photoreceptor protein renewal in early retinal reattachment. *Am J Ophthalmol* 1971;72:356–366.

Marcus DF, Aaberg TM: Intraretinal macrocysts in retinal detachment. *Arch Ophthalmol* 1979;97:1273–1275.

Michels RG, Wilkinson CP, Rice TA: *Retinal Detachment.* St Louis: CV Mosby Co; 1990.

Norton EWD: Retinal detachment in aphakia. *Trans Am Ophthalmol Soc* 1963;61:770–789.

Okun E: Histopathology of changes which precede retinal detachment. *Bibl Ophthalmol* 1966;70:76–97.

O'Malley P, Allen RA, Straatsma BR, et al: Paving-stone degeneration of the retina. *Arch Ophthalmol* 1965;73:169–182.

Retina Society Terminology Committee. The classification of retinal detachment with proliferative vitreoretinopathy. *Ophthalmology* 1983;90:121–125.

Robertson DM, Curtin VT, Norton EWD: Avulsed retinal vessels with retinal breaks: a cause of recurrent vitreous hemorrhage. *Arch Ophthalmol* 1971;85:669–672.

Rutnin U, Schepens CL: Fundus appearance in normal eyes. *Am J Ophthalmol* 1967;64: 821–852, 1040–1078.

Ryan SJ: Traction retinal detachment. XLIX Edward Jackson Memorial Lecture. *Am J Ophthalmol* 1993;115:1–20.

Schepens CL: Diagnostic and prognostic factors as found in preoperative examination. *Trans Am Acad Ophthalmol Otolaryngol* 1952;56:398–412.

Sigelman J: Vitreous base classification of retinal tears: clinical application. *Surv Ophthalmol* 1980;25:59–70.

Smiddy WE, Green WR: Retinal dialysis: pathology and pathogenesis. *Retina* 1982;2: 94–116.

Straatsma BR, Foos RY: Typical and reticular degenerative retinoschisis. XXVI Francis I. Proctor Memorial Lecture. *Am J Ophthalmol* 1973;75:551–575.

Straatsma BR, Zeegen PD, Foos RY, et al: Lattice degeneration of the retina. XXX Edward Jackson Memorial Lecture. *Trans Am Acad Ophthalmol Otolaryngol* 1974;78:OP87–113.

Tani P, Robertson DM, Langworthy A: Rhegmatogenous retinal detachment without macular involvement treated with scleral buckling. *Am J Ophthalmol* 1980;90:503–508.

Tasman W: Retinal detachment with breaks in the pars plana. *Br J Ophthalmol* 1968;52: 181–183.

Wallyn RH, Hilton GF: Subretinal fibrosis in retinal detachment. *Arch Ophthalmol* 1979;97: 2128–2129.

CHAPTER 3

Preoperative Examination

The preoperative examination of the patient consists principally of history taking, measurement of visual acuity, external examination, ocular motility testing, testing of pupillary reactions, biomicroscopy, tonometry, and binocular indirect ophthalmoscopy. Contact-lens biomicroscopy, perimetry, and ultrasonography are also sometimes required.

3-1 HISTORY

The symptoms of retinal detachment include flashes of light, floaters, visual field defect, decreased visual acuity, metamorphopsia, and, very rarely, defective color vision.

3-1-1 Flashes of Light

The perception of light flashes, or photopsia, is due to the production of phosphenes by pathophysiologic stimulus of the retina. The retina is stimulated by light but is also capable of responding to mechanical disturbances. In fact, the most common cause of light flashes is posterior vitreous detachment. As the vitreous separates from the retinal surface, the retina is disturbed mechanically, stimulating a sensation of light. This perception is more marked if there are focal vitreoretinal adhesions. Generally, vitreous separation is benign and may almost be regarded as normal in the senescent eye. In approximately 12% of symptomatic posterior vitreous detachments, however, a careful search of the periphery reveals a tear of the retina.

If the flashes are associated with floaters, it is wise to assume that a retinal tear exists until proved otherwise. These symptoms demand a careful examination of the periphery with binocular indirect ophthalmoscopy and scleral indentation. The patient's localization of the photopsia is of no value in predicting the location of the vitreoretinal pathology. If no breaks are evident in the first examination after symptomatic vitreous detachment, they rarely appear at a later date.

If there is no associated hemorrhage or other pathologic condition, the patient needs counseling only. However, if pigment or blood is detected in the vitreous, followup examination is required. It is prudent to forewarn patients about the symptoms of retinal detachment. Flashes alone or floaters alone are less significant than if they occur together, in which case they are more likely to be associated with a retinal break.

The light scintillations of ocular migraine are correctly identified by the typical history. However, ophthalmoscopic examination is required to rule out a retinal cause.

3-1-2 Floaters

While a few floaters (muscae volitantes) are experienced almost universally by the general population, the acute onset of new floaters requires careful examination. A patient describing hundreds of tiny black specks is virtually pathognomonic of vitreous hemorrhage. The sudden appearance of one large floater near the visual axis is ordinarily caused by posterior vitreous separation in which the glial annulus (Weiss' ring) of the posterior vitreous has pulled loose from its peripapillary location. The appearance of numerous curvilinear opacities within the visual field generally indicates vitreous degeneration. Small vitreous collagen fibrils resulting from degeneration coalesce into large, coarse fibers, which cast curvilinear shadows on the retina.

The most significant cause of floaters is vitreous hemorrhage, and the characteristic numerous tiny black dots may be followed in a few hours by "cobwebs" as the blood forms irregular clots. The cause of acute vitreous hemorrhage must be assumed to be a retinal tear until proved otherwise. If the entire fundus cannot be adequately visualized, examination by ultrasonography is recommended. If a retinal detachment is found, the eye should be managed with vitrectomy. Otherwise, the patient should be kept in a sitting position with both eyes patched for at least 48 hours to allow settling of the blood. This approach may produce sufficient clearing to reveal the presence of a retinal break that can be treated.

3-1-3 Visual Field Defects

Awareness by the patient of a visual field defect or shadow is the first symptom of retinal detachment. Detachments anterior to the equator have no effect on the visual field and cannot be demonstrated with perimetry. Detachments posterior to the equator can be demonstrated by perimetry, but patients rarely notice a field defect until the detachment encroaches on the posterior pole. Patients tend to be less aware of superior than inferior field defects, and those patients with inferior retinal detachments may be totally unaware of superior field loss until the fovea is involved. High bullous detachments cause dense field defects; flat detachments produce relative field defects.

Light flashes and floaters have no value for localization of retinal breaks, but visual field examination is highly specific for localizing retinal detachments. When a patient with extensive retinal detachment is being examined, it is frequently helpful to inquire about the position of the field defect when first seen as a clue to the location of the primary retinal break. For instance, if a patient with a total retinal detachment has a history of an inferior nasal field defect that later enlarged to involve the total field, the finding of a retinal break in the superior temporal periphery is likely.

3-1-4 Decreased Central Acuity

Although the duration of retinal detachment symptoms is estimated from the time of the onset of the visual field defect, the duration of foveal involvement dates from the time of decreased central acuity. The prognosis for recovery of central vision is approximately correlated with the duration of foveal detachment. Peripheral field loss may escape a patient's notice, so that medical help is not sought until central vision is lost.

3-1-5 Trauma

The patient should be queried about a history of trauma, either accidental or surgical. The examiner should carefully record the details of trauma in the patient's chart, remembering that it is a legal document that might later be reviewed. The time, place, and nature of the accident should be entered. Direct trauma to the globe should be clearly differentiated from any indirect trauma to the head or elsewhere in the body. Details of previous surgery should be noted, particularly cataract extraction, intraocular foreign body removal, and retinal procedures. Frequently, a patient denies any trauma during the initial examination but recalls some remote trauma a few weeks later. The denial and the recollection should be recorded under the date that each is reported by the patient.

3-1-6 Ocular Diseases

The history must include questions regarding previous ocular diseases, such as uveitis, vitreous hemorrhage, amblyopia, glaucoma, or diabetic retinopathy. Any symptom of retinal detachment can be mimicked by other disease processes. Light flashes might be due to posterior vitreous detachment, floaters to age-related vitreous degeneration or uveitis, quadrantic field defects to occlusion of a branch of the central retinal artery, and loss of the entire visual field to occlusion of one of the central vessels or to massive vitreous hemorrhage.

3-1-7 Systemic Diseases

A careful history of the patient's general health includes specific questions about systemic disorders that are sometimes associated with retinal detachment, including diabetes, tumors, angiomatosis of the central nervous system, sickle cell disease, leukemia, and eclampsia.

3-1-8 Family History

Although most retinal detachments occur as sporadic events, certain families are susceptible to retinal detachment. A family history of retinal detachment is a clue to prognosis and frequently indicates the need for examination of other family members. The history influences decisions regarding prophylactic treatment of retinal breaks.

3-2

VISUAL ACUITY

The best corrected visual acuity should be recorded for each eye. Generally, the patient's current eyeglasses or contact lenses suffice, but if there is any doubt, a refraction should be done. Visual acuity is usually measured with the Snellen test. Low vision may be recorded with a decreasing numerator of the Snellen fraction, such as 5/200 or 2/200. Because the examiner's fingers are grossly equivalent to the 20/200 letter, counting fingers at a distance of 5 feet is approximately equivalent to 5/200. The visual acuity of illiterate or non–English-speaking patients or of preliterate children can be measured with the E chart.

Decreased visual acuity always accompanies extension of the retinal detachment into the fovea, but it does not necessarily mean detachment of the fovea. Poor central vision may also be due to antecedent disease of the macula, opacities of the media, optic nerve disease, or amblyopia.

3-3

EXTERNAL EXAMINATION

The examiner should record the status of the brows, lashes, and lids. Accurate recording of the preoperative state of these structures is a requisite base for postoperative evaluation of the external anatomy. The early postoperative period may be characterized by pseudoptosis, lid edema, chemosis, and, rarely, permanent ptosis.

3-4

OCULAR MOTILITY

Retinal reattachment surgery is occasionally accompanied by temporary changes in the function of the extraocular muscles, and in rare cases the changes are permanent. Therefore, a preoperative record of the state of ocular motility is mandatory. Although there are many tests of motility, the cover test and versions usually suffice. But when the vision of one or both eyes is poor, the cover test is not reliable. In such a case, the examiner should simply note the position of the light reflection of the flashlight with reference to the visual axis of each cornea (Hirschberg test). Each millimeter deviation of the corneal light reflex from the visual axis is equivalent to approximately 12 prism diopters (Δ). This test can be refined by selection of the appropriate prism to restore the light reflex to the normal visual axis (Krimsky test).

3-5

PERIMETRY

Most cases of retinal detachment can be evaluated adequately without perimetry, but there are certain instances in which it is helpful and others in which it is mandatory. The visual fields should be examined by confrontation, and if there is any question about the correlation of the field defect with the detachment, formal perimetry should be performed. Perimetry is always indicated if there is antecedent disease of the optic nerve, particularly glaucomatous cupping.

Perimetry may also be helpful in the differential diagnosis of retinoschisis. Relatively flat retinoschisis can be readily differentiated from shallow retinal detachment, in that the former invariably causes an absolute field defect while the latter causes only a relative defect. Perimetry is less specific for bullous detachment, because an absolute field defect could be found in either detachment or retinoschisis. Perimetry may be helpful with a miotic pupil, which occasionally is the first sign of detachment in a patient having miotic treatment for glaucoma. As previously mentioned, perimetry only discloses disease posterior to the equator.

3-6

PUPILLARY REACTIONS

Pupillary reactions should be noted, and the size of the maximally dilated pupil recorded. Subtle differences in the direct light reflex might not be apparent unless a comparison is made between the two eyes with a swinging flashlight (Marcus Gunn test), by which the direct pupillary reflex is studied in contrast to the consensual reflex. A test is positive when the pupil dilates as the light is directed into it, indicating that the direct reflex is weaker than the consensual. Any defect in the afferent pupillomotor system, including retinal detachment, results in a positive test and is referred to as an *afferent pupillary defect.*

3-7

BIOMICROSCOPY

The cornea is usually clear in retinal detachment, but occasionally there is enough hypotony to create folds in Descemet's membrane. Anterior uveitis is rarely sufficient to produce keratic precipitates. Mild flare and cells are frequently noted in the anterior chamber, and occasionally the reaction is marked. The depth of the anterior chamber should be noted. The angle of the chamber can be estimated with the slit-lamp beam near the limbus. This assessment usually suffices, but if the results are unclear, gonioscopy is indicated.

A normal lens, as well as any opacities of the lens, should be noted. An objective assessment of the effect of opacities on visual acuity is more accurate with use of the direct ophthalmoscope. A posterior subcapsular cataract might interfere with visual acuity, but it does not prevent a thorough examination of the fundus periphery. On the other hand, peripheral cortical opacities may not interfere with visual acuity, but they may seriously impair examination of the periphery and conceal the presence of peripheral retinal breaks. The vitreous should be examined for evidence of vitreous detachment, hemorrhage, inflammatory cells, or pigment.

If there has been no previous intraocular disturbance, such as uveitis, trauma, or intraocular surgery, the presence of pigment in the vitreous ("tobacco dust") is very suggestive of a retinal break. If a retinal break allows contact between the vitreous and the pigment epithelium, shedding of pigment through the break into the vitreous cavity occurs. Retinal breaks have been found in more than 70% of eyes with "tobacco dust" if there is no other obvious explanation for the presence of pigment in the vitreous.

3-8

TONOMETRY

The intraocular tension should be recorded for both eyes before the pressure is artificially lowered by the massage effect of scleral indentation (scleral depression). Usually, an eye with retinal detachment is relatively hypotonic, and the pressure may be as much as 10 mm Hg less than the unaffected eye. Occasionally, the hypotony is so profound that no tension can be recorded. Still rarer is the patient who has a paradoxically elevated intraocular pressure in the presence of retinal detachment (Schwartz syndrome). Either of these extremes is usually relieved by retinal reattachment.

3-9

BINOCULAR INDIRECT OPHTHALMOSCOPY

Most retinal surgeons rely primarily on the binocular indirect ophthalmoscope. Its main features are contrasted with those of the direct ophthalmoscope in Table 3-1. Despite the inverted and reversed image, the binocular indirect ophthalmoscope has been widely accepted due to its large field, high illumination, depth of focus, stereopsis, and especially its ease of use with the scleral indentor.

Scleral indentation is helpful in bringing the far periphery of the retina into view, but its greatest advantage is that the retina can be seen in tangential profile. As the examiner indents the peripheral retina, minute changes of retinal contour are readily demonstrated. The technique enables visualization of a retinal flap as it rises from the crest of the indentor mound (Figure 3-1). A red spot might be shown to be a hemorrhage on the surface of the retina, instead of a retinal hole; an ill-defined gray area might be revealed as an excavation; a white spot might turn out to be a tuft of tissue rising from the retinal surface; and so on. Mastery of the binocular indirect ophthalmoscope requires many hours of effort, and instruction in its use is best obtained from an instructor endowed with great patience. (For further discussion of ophthalmoscopic technique, see the appendix.)

When several physicians must share an ophthalmoscope, an instrument with an adjustable headband and interpupillary distance is recommended. An individual examiner may prefer a spectacle-mounted ophthalmoscope because of its lighter weight and portability. Equipped with a rechargeable power pack, the latter is particularly useful for rounds and surgery.

Many condensing lenses can be used for indirect ophthalmoscopy, but the most popular is the +20 D lens with aspheric curves and a diameter of 50 mm. Lenses with greater power afford a larger field of view but less magnification, and lenses with less power have a smaller field of view but greater magnification. While the indirect ophthalmoscope is usually used at arm's length, increased magnification of a specific lesion can be obtained by examination at a closer working distance. A greater distance, with the elbows fully extended, is a definite advantage when examining a patient with small pupils. The indirect ophthalmoscope is also useful for examining the anterior segment of in-

TABLE 3-1

Features of Direct vs Binocular Indirect Ophthalmoscopy

Feature	Direct	Indirect (+20 lens)
Magnification	14×	3×
Field diameter	2 DD	9 DD
Ratio of area of field	1	20
Illumination	Limited	High
Depth of focus	Small	Large
Stereopsis	Absent	Present
Orientation of image	Direct	Inverted, reversed
View of periphery	Limited	Full
Working distance	Close	Arm's length
Scleral indentation	Difficult	Easy

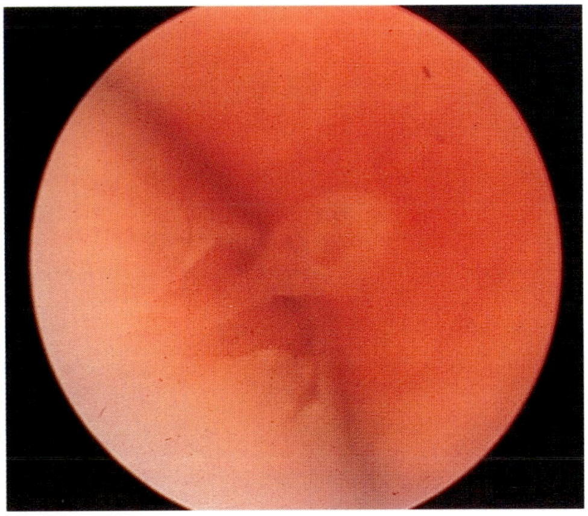

Figure 3-1 *Flap of retinal tear, clearly seen as it arises from crest of mound created by scleral indentor.*

Reproduced with permission of Medcom, Inc., from Conor O'Malley, MD, FACS, and Patrick O'Malley, MD, FACS: "The Peripheral Fundus of the Eye."

TABLE 3-2

Color Code for Fundus Chart

Color	Finding
Black	1 Retinal or choroidal hyperpigmentation
	2 Fibrous proliferation
	3 Cotton-wool patch
	4 Ora serrata
	5 Exudate
	6 Drusen
Blue	1 Detached retina
	2 Retinoschisis
	3 Lattice
	4 Veins
Yellow	Label specific lesion, eg, recent treatment with diathermy or photocoagulation, active chorioretinitis, retinal edema
Brown	Pigment under detached retina
White	Normal attached retina
Green	Opacities of media; label specific lesion, eg, cataract, vitreous hemorrhage, or corneal opacity
Purple	Flat neovascularization
Orange	Elevated neovascularization
Red	1 Retinal breaks
	2 Thin retina
	3 Preretinal, intraretinal, and subretinal hemorrhages
	4 Microaneurysms
	5 Arteries

patients when the examiner's eyes are positioned just 8 to 10 inches from the patient and the condensing lens functions as a magnifying loupe that provides an erect real image.

Much of the retinal surface can be examined with the patient in the seated position, but most surgeons prefer to place the patient in the supine position. If the examiner wants to check for shifting subretinal fluid, unroll the flap of a superior giant break, or shift an overhanging superior bulla to gain a view of the fovea, it is helpful to position the supine patient's head over the edge of the table. By marked hyperextension of the neck, the patient can be placed in a head-down position. This positioning technique often yields valuable information.

The details of the detached retina should be drawn on a large fundus chart, which consists of three concentric circles representing the equator, the ora serrata, and the anterior limit of the pars plana (Figure 3-2). An inherent misrepresentation in the chart results from reduction of the three-dimensional eye to a two-dimensional drawing. Colored pencils are used to record the findings according to the code described in Table 3-2.

Examination of a large number of fundi has revealed certain hemiretinal differences. The temporal periphery is the most common site of lattice degeneration, retinal breaks, pars plana cysts, dialysis of the young, and degenerative retinoschisis. The nasal periphery is the most common site of prominent ora teeth, meridional folds at the ora, granular tissue, and detachment of the pars plana.

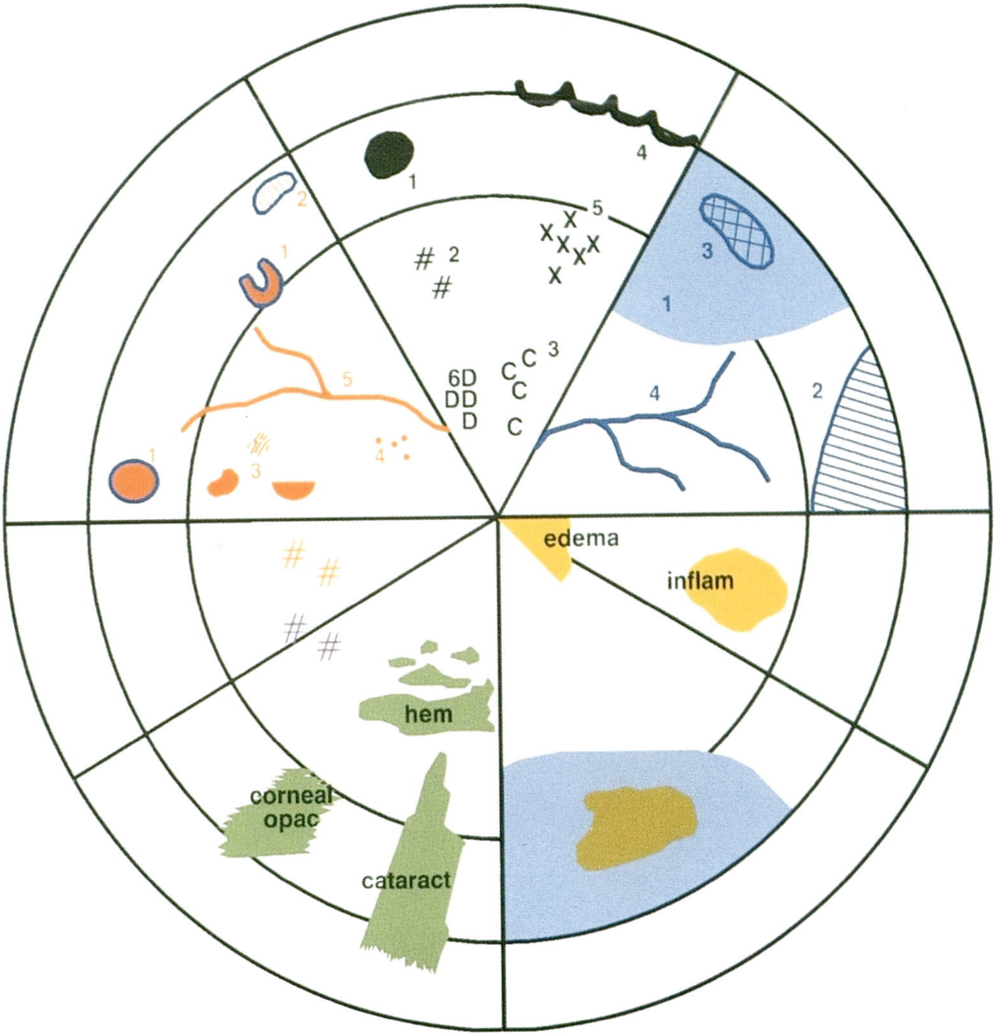

Figure 3-2 *Fundus chart illustrating potential details of a detached retina recorded in colored pencil. Table 3-2 describes color code.*

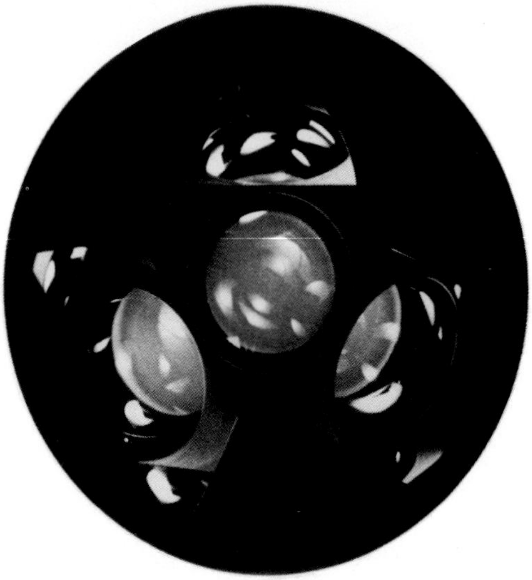

Figure 3-3 *Goldmann three-mirror lens.*
Reproduced with permission from Cockerham WD, Schepens CL: Technique of vitreous cavity examination. In: Symposium on Retina and Retinal Surgery *(Transactions of the New Orleans Academy of Ophthalmology). St Louis: CV Mosby Co; 1969: 66–89.*

3-10

CONTACT-LENS BIOMICROSCOPY

Biomicroscopic examination of the posterior segment is accomplished by the use of a flat, macular, three-mirror, or four-mirror contact lens (Figures 3-3, 3-4). The biomicroscope provides stereopsis, high illumination, high magnification, and the great advantage of a slit-beam optical section. Routine use of diagnostic contact lenses is not required for every retinal detachment, but in selected cases they reveal valuable information not obtainable by any other method.

Through the flat central portion of the lens, it is possible to examine the central and posterior vitreous. There is no better way to examine the optic nerve head and the fine details of macular anatomy. The technique is particularly valuable in the search for posterior retinal breaks, which are particularly difficult to locate in the staphyloma of highly myopic eyes or in the retinal detachment of proliferative diabetic retinopathy. Vitreoretinal relationships in the periphery can be examined with the larger mirrors. The smallest mirror is valuable for examining the ora serrata and the anterior chamber angle. It is a simple matter to include observation of the angle with contact-lens examination of the fundus periphery. One advantage of this examination is the shallow depth of focus, which is valuable when a questionable retinal break cannot be clearly defined by ophthalmoscopy. By precise focus on the sensory retina, the presence of a break can be detected.

Biomicroscopy is the best way to define the critical role of the detached vitreous cortex in proliferative diabetic retinopathy. The mechanism of elevation of previously flat neovascularization, avulsion of retinal vessels, and tractional retinal detachment can be clearly seen.

Biomicroscopy is also valuable for the preoperative evaluation of a patient with a giant retinal tear. The possible attachment of formed vitreous to the flap of the tear or the presence of formed vitreous behind the retina is a preoperative clue to the prognosis and suggests the best technique of surgical management.

Binocular indirect ophthalmoscopy should be employed first to obtain a panoramic view of the entire posterior segment. Contact-lens biomicroscopy can then be used to define specific details; that is, the indirect ophthalmoscope can be used to see the "forest," and the slit lamp to see the individual "trees." Exclusive reliance on slit-lamp examination of the retina is not recommended.

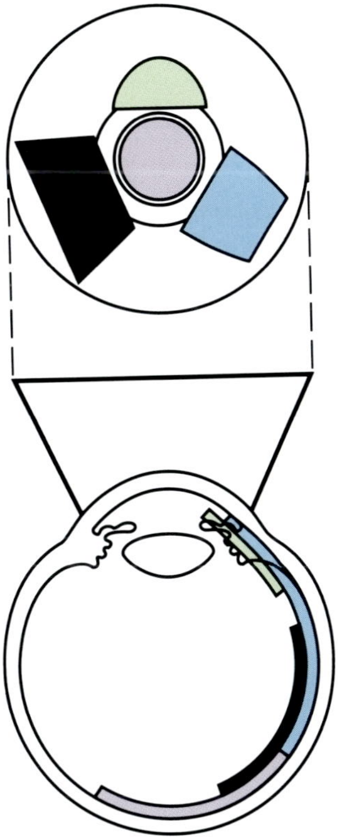

Figure 3-4 *Diagram of fundus areas visible with Goldmann three-mirror lens.*

Redrawn with permission from Havener WH, Gloeckner S: Atlas of Diagnostic Techniques and Treatment of Retinal Detachment. *St Louis: CV Mosby Co; 1967.*

3-11

ULTRASONOGRAPHY

When confronted with opaque media, the physician can obtain valuable information with ultrasonography—both A-scan and B-scan. The technique can reveal both rhegmatogenous and nonrhegmatogenous detachments, such as those secondary to malignant melanoma of the choroid (Figure 3-5).

Figure 3-5 *Ultrasonograms. (A) Rhegmatogenous detachment. (B) Detachment secondary to malignant melanoma.*

Reproduced with permission from Coleman DJ, Jack RL: B-scan ultrasonography in diagnosis and management of retinal detachments. Arch Ophthalmol *1973;90:29–34. Copyright 1973 American Medical Association.*

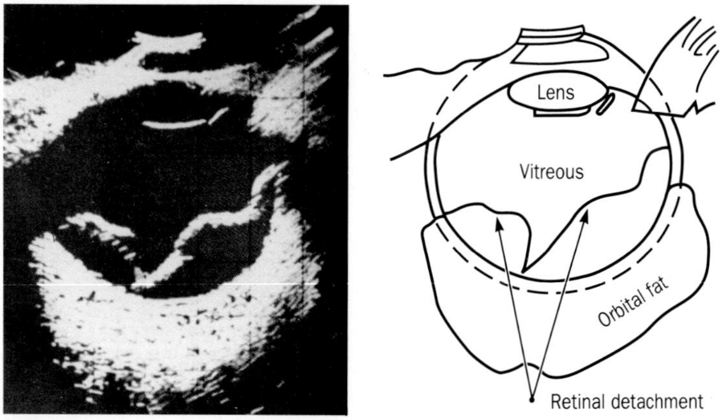

A

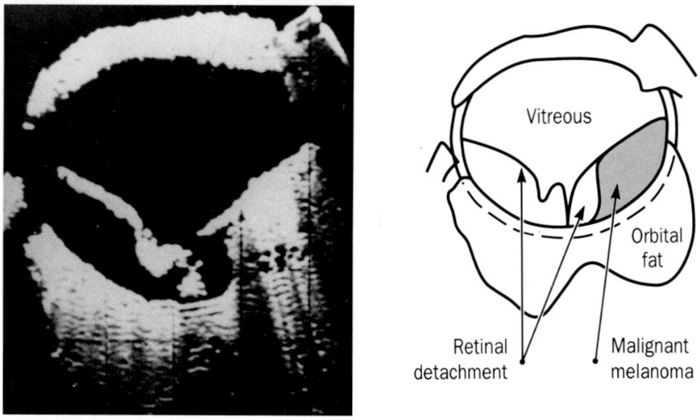

B

3-12

FUNDUS CHANGES INSIGNIFICANT TO DETACHMENT

The most prominent feature of the fundus is the optic nerve head or disc, the only place in the human body that affords a direct view of a tract of the central nervous system. The foveola, the functional center of the fundus, is located in the center of the fovea, which has a diameter of about 5°. The macula is centered on the fovea and has a diameter of about 17°. The multiple branches of the central retinal artery are readily identified by their bright red color and relatively narrow caliber. The multiple tributaries of the central retinal vein are recognized by their dark red color and relatively wider caliber.

In a darkly pigmented fundus, the choroidal vessels in the posterior pole can be

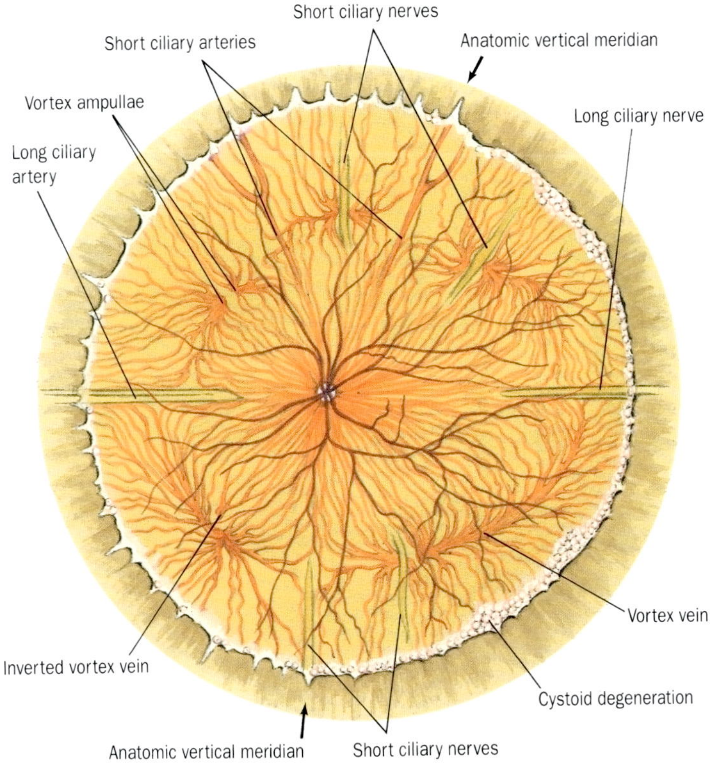

Figure 3-6 *Normal fundus. with principal structures labeled.*
Reproduced from Rutnin U, Schepens CL: Fundus appearance in normal eyes. Am J Ophthalmol *1967;64:821–852, 1040–1078. Published with permission from The American Journal of Ophthalmology. Copyright by The Ophthalmic Publishing Company.*

obscured from view; but in an eye with minimal pigment, they are readily visible. The venous tributaries of the choroid that make up the vortex veins are usually easily seen. The most prominent features of the choroidal venous system are the vortex ampullae, of which there are usually four but sometimes more. They are located approximately in the 1-, 5-, 7-, and 11-o'clock meridians, just posterior to the equator. The horizontal meridians are usually identifiable by their radially oriented, long posterior ciliary nerves, and infrequently the long posterior ciliary artery can be seen adjacent to the nerve. The nerve is relatively broad and has a yellow color, and the artery is identifiable by its red color. The artery is usually inferior to the nerve temporally and superior to it nasally (Figure 3-6).

The ora serrata is the anterior limit of the sensory retina. It is characterized nasally by prominent ora teeth, which point anteriorly. Between each pair of teeth is an ora bay (Figures 3-7, 3-8). The pattern of serration is not present temporally, where the ora teeth are small or absent (Figure 3-9). There are approximately 48 teeth per eye. Occasionally, a white line is

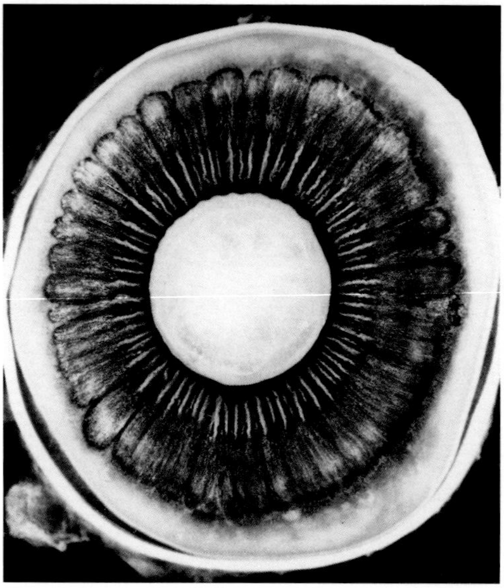

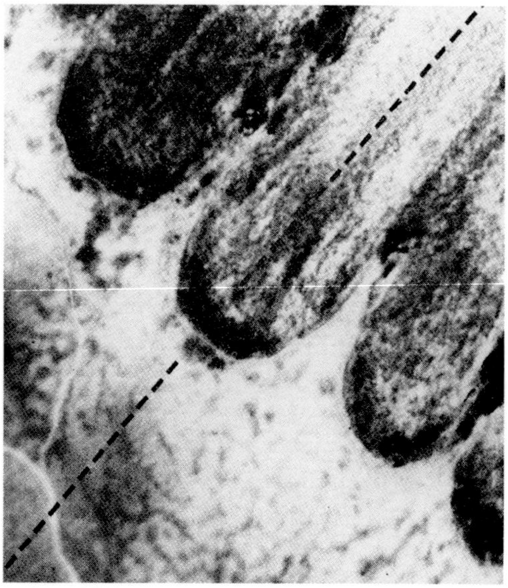

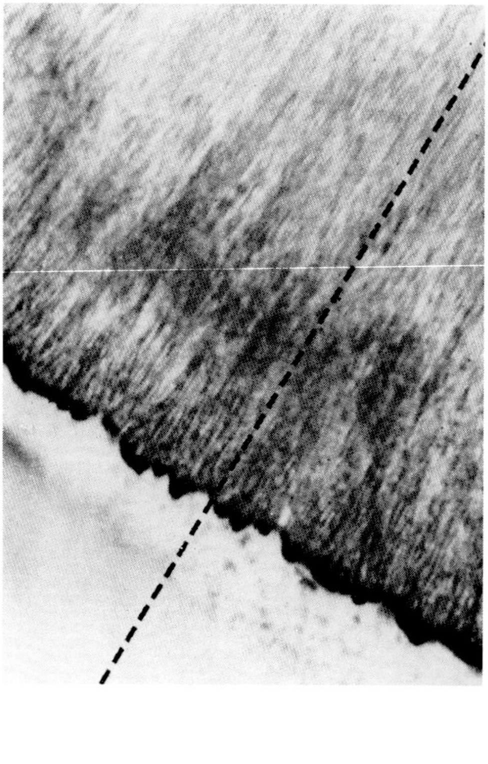

Figure 3-7 *Autopsy photograph of ora serrata and ciliary body.*

Reproduced with permission from Straatsma BR, Foos RY, Spencer LM: The retina—topography and clinical correlations. In: Symposium on Retina and Retinal Surgery *(Transactions of the New Orleans Academy of Ophthalmology). St Louis: CV Mosby Co; 1969:1–26.*

Figure 3-8 *(Top right) Autopsy photograph of nasal ora serrata.*

Reproduced with permission from Straatsma BR, et al: The Retina: Morphology, Function, and Clinical Characteristics. *UCLA Forum in Medical Sciences, No. 8. Copyright © 1969 The Regents of the University of California.*

Figure 3-9 *(Right) Autopsy photograph of temporal ora serrata.*

Reproduced with permission from Straatsma BR, et al: The Retina: Morphology, Function, and Clinical Characteristics. *UCLA Forum in Medical Sciences, No. 8. Copyright © 1969 The Regents of the University of California.*

evident on the retina just posterior to the ora serrata, representing the posterior limit of the vitreous base (see Figure 2-22). A similar circumferential white line representing the anterior limit of the vitreous base is occasionally visible in the middle of the pars plana.

The normal fusion of the sensory retina and retinal pigment epithelium along the ora serrata is referred to as the *retinochoroidal adhesion*. This zone is 3 or 4 mm wide in the temporal periphery but less than 1 mm wide in the nasal periphery. It is pigmented, a feature easily demonstrated by transillumination. The anterior progression of a retinal detachment is generally halted by this adhesion, but occasionally the subretinal fluid breaks through to create detachment of the pars plana, in which there is separation of the nonpigmented and pigmented epithelial layers. Detachment of the pars plana, sometimes called *detachment of the ora*, is more common on the nasal side, apparently because of the narrower retinochoroidal adhesion. Detachment of the pars plana epithelium is an important feature, and the pars plana must be carefully examined with scleral indentation to detect the presence of breaks in the area, particularly along the anterior limit of the vitreous base.

The periphery of the fundus extends from the equator to the anterior limit of the pars plana, constituting about one third of the total fundus. It is the most important area as far as detachment-producing lesions are concerned.

The equator is an important landmark for the recording of retinal findings, but the beginning ophthalmoscopist might have difficulty identifying it. It is helpful to recall that the distance from the ora to the equator is approximately 4 disc diameters and that the equator is just slightly anterior to the vortex ampullae.

Proceeding forward from the tip of an ora tooth, the examiner may find a faint line extending anteriorly into the corresponding valley of the pars plicata. Such lines are known as *striae ciliares*. The transition axis between the deep nasal ora bays and the shallow temporal bays is a line that extends approximately from the 11- to the 5-o'clock position in the right eye and from the 1- to the 7-o'clock position in the left. A fold of redundant retina is commonly associated with the ora teeth, particularly in the superior nasal quadrant. Often found in an ora bay, these meridional folds are usually benign, but occasionally there is an associated retinal break, in most instances at the posterior limit of the fold.

Variations of the morphology of ora teeth include forked teeth, bridging teeth, giant teeth, and ring-shaped teeth (Figure 3-10). Occasionally, an ora bay is surrounded by retinal tissue, and such an enclosed bay must be differentiated from a true retinal break, which it mimics (Figure 3-11). Sometimes, a deep ora bay is seen nasally at the horizontal meridian. A dense, shiny-white spherical structure is sometimes seen near the ora serrata. Known as an *ora pearl*, it has no clinical significance despite its remarkable appearance (Figure 3-12A).

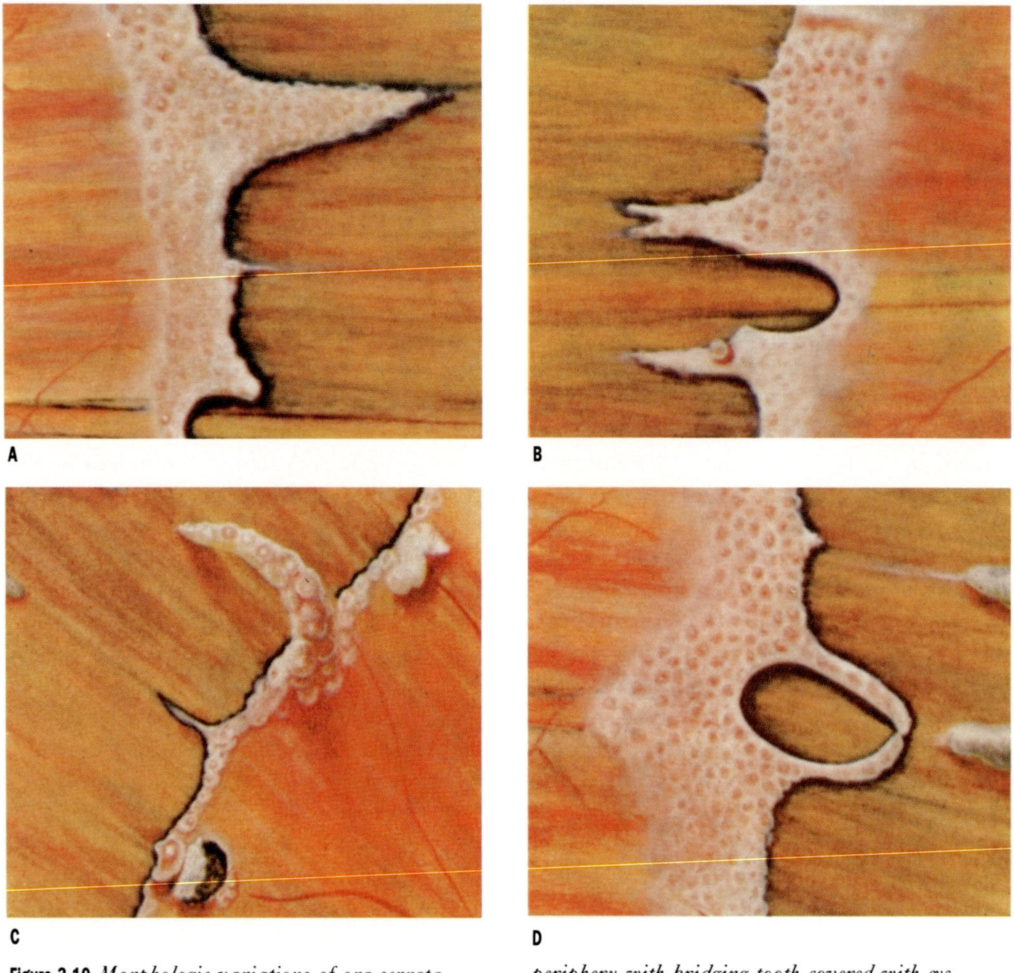

Figure 3-10 *Morphologic variations of ora serrata region in normal fundi. (A) Nasal periphery with marked cystoid degeneration near horizontal meridian, giant tooth, and deep ora bay over long ciliary nerve. (B) Temporal periphery with marked cystoid degeneration near horizontal meridian, deep ora bay over long ciliary nerve, with forked tooth (above) and tooth with pearl at its base (below). Second pearl is visible at anterior end of inferior tooth; small meridional fold on side of ora bay (above). (C) Upper temporal periphery with bridging tooth covered with cystoid degeneration and almost in contact with ciliary process; granular globule (above) and white granular patch with large cystoid cavity on its anterior border (below). (D) Nasal periphery near horizontal meridian, with marked cystoid degeneration; ring tooth (closed ring) over long ciliary nerve; small meridional fold over ora tooth (below). (E) Temporal periphery near horizontal meridian; deep ora bay over long ciliary nerve; tooth above deep bay had part of tip bro-*

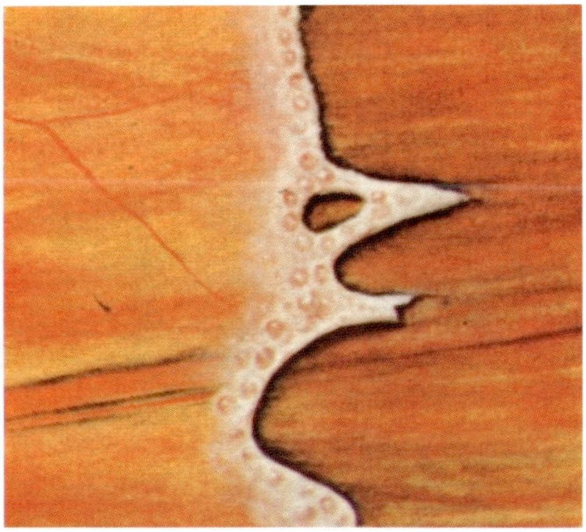

E

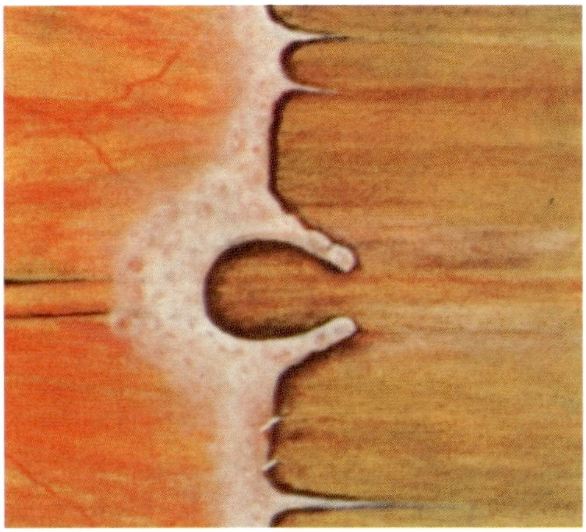

F

ken off; ring tooth (hole-in-the-tooth; above). (F) Nasal periphery, near horizontal meridian, with ring tooth (open ring) and deep ora bay over long ciliary nerve. In next bay (below), two tiny tags.

Reproduced from Rutnin U, Schepens CL: Fundus appearance in normal eyes. Am J Ophthalmol *1967; 64:821–852, 1040–1078. Published with permission from The American Journal of Ophthalmology. Copyright by The Ophthalmic Publishing Company.*

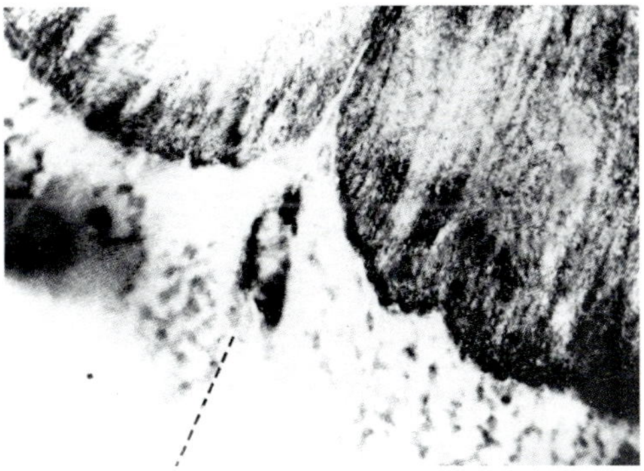

Figure 3-11 *Autopsy photograph of enclosed ora bay. Reproduced with permission from Straatsma BR, et al:* The Retina: Morphology, Function, and Clinical Characteristics. *UCLA Forum in Medical Sciences, No. 8. Copyright © 1969 The Regents of the University of California.*

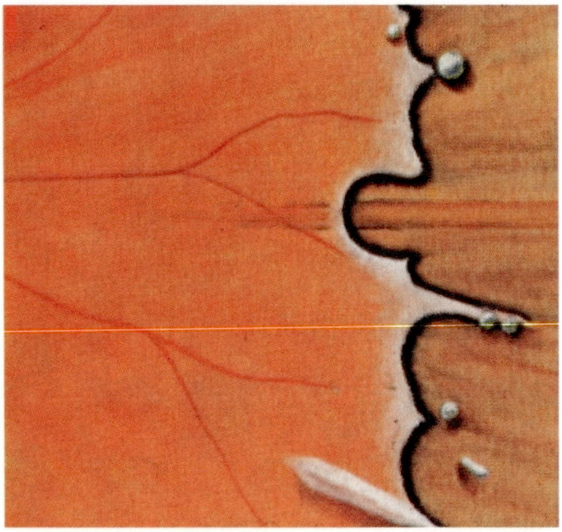

A

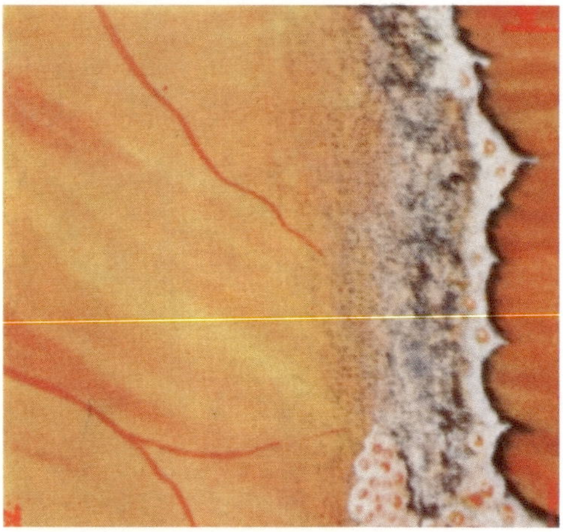

B

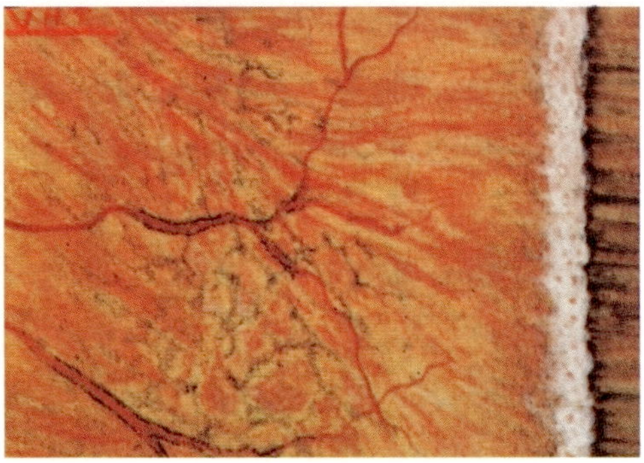

C

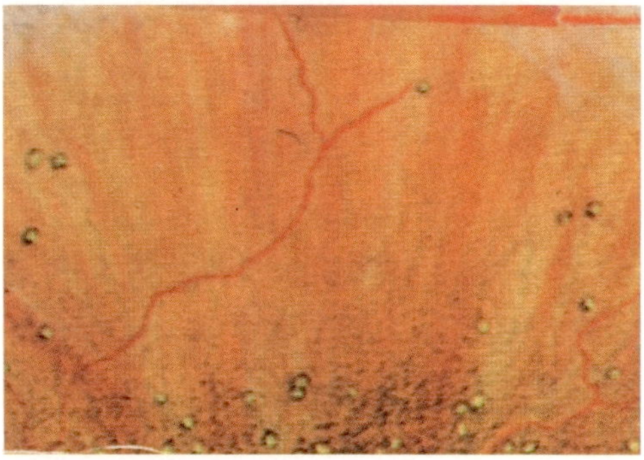

D

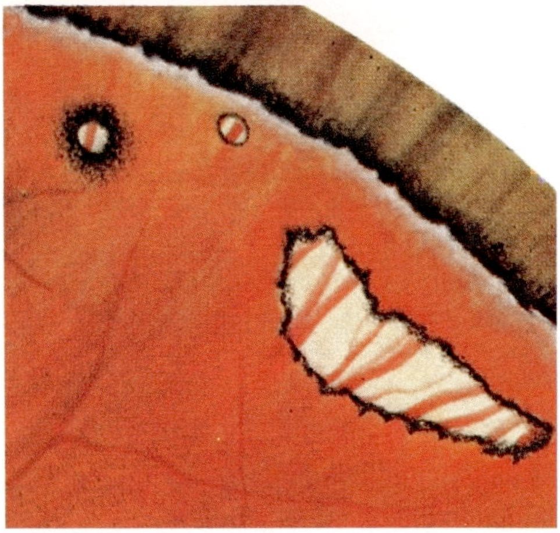

E

Figure 3-12 *Changes of fundus periphery thought to be clinically insignificant. (A) Composite picture of temporal periphery shows size, shape, and location of pearls. (B) Chorioretinal degeneration at ora serrata. (C) Reticular pigmentary degeneration at equator. (D) Equatorial drusen. (E) Paving-stone degeneration. (F) White with/without pressure. (G) Composite painting illustrating sizes and shapes of pars plana cysts. (H) Retinal erosion.*

Reproduced from Rutnin U, Schepens CL: Fundus appearance in normal eyes. Am J Ophthalmol *1967; 64:821–852, 1040–1078. Published with permission from The American Journal of Ophthalmology. Copyright by The Ophthalmic Publishing Company.*

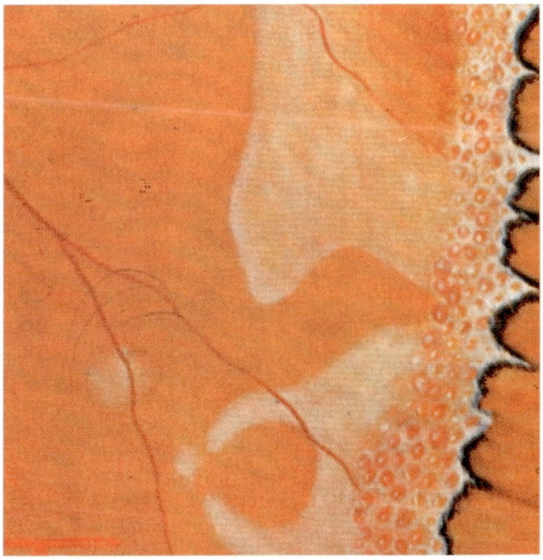

F

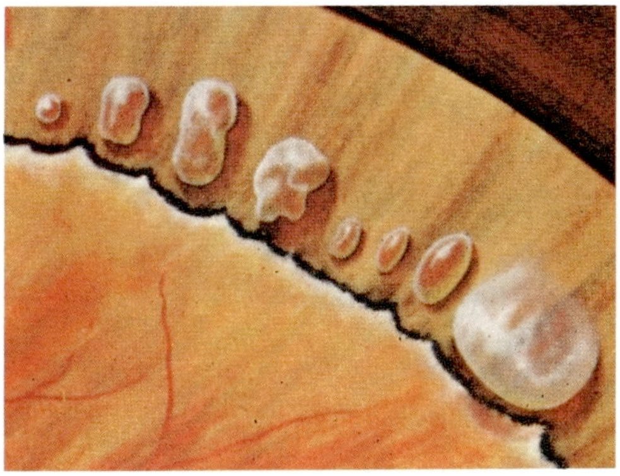

G

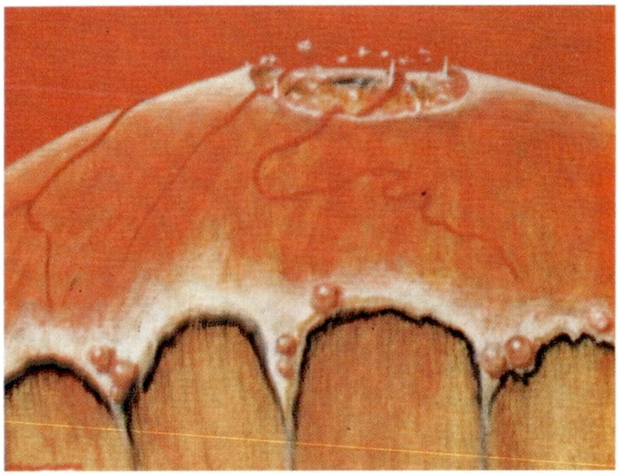

H

Tufts of redundant glial tissue at or near the ora are called *cystic retinal tufts* but also have been termed *congenital retinal rosettes*, *glial spheres*, and *granular tissue* (Figures 3-13 to 3-15). Rarely, an elevated tuft of retinal tissue points toward the anterior segment. This malformation is due to traction from a zonule and is therefore called a *zonular traction tuft*. Changes in the fundus thought to be clinically insignificant in the production of retinal detachment include chorioretinal degeneration near the ora, reticular pigmentary degeneration, equatorial drusen, paving-stone degeneration, whitening of the retina, pars plana cysts, retinal erosion, and pigment clumps (see Figure 3-12).

3-12-1 Chorioretinal Degeneration

Chorioretinal degeneration is the term for a stippled salt-and-pepper type of pigment alteration that often occurs adjacent to the ora. Infrequently, degeneration is also found more posteriorly toward the equator and, when located between the ora and the equator, it apparently halts the posterior progression of more anteriorly located peripheral cystoid degeneration (see Figure 3-12B).

3-12-2 Reticular Pigmentary Degeneration

This condition occurs in the aging eye, and the frequency increases with advancing age. Also called *honeycomb chorioretinal degeneration*, it is caused by retinal pigment epithelial degeneration and is most prominent along the nasal equator. The pig-

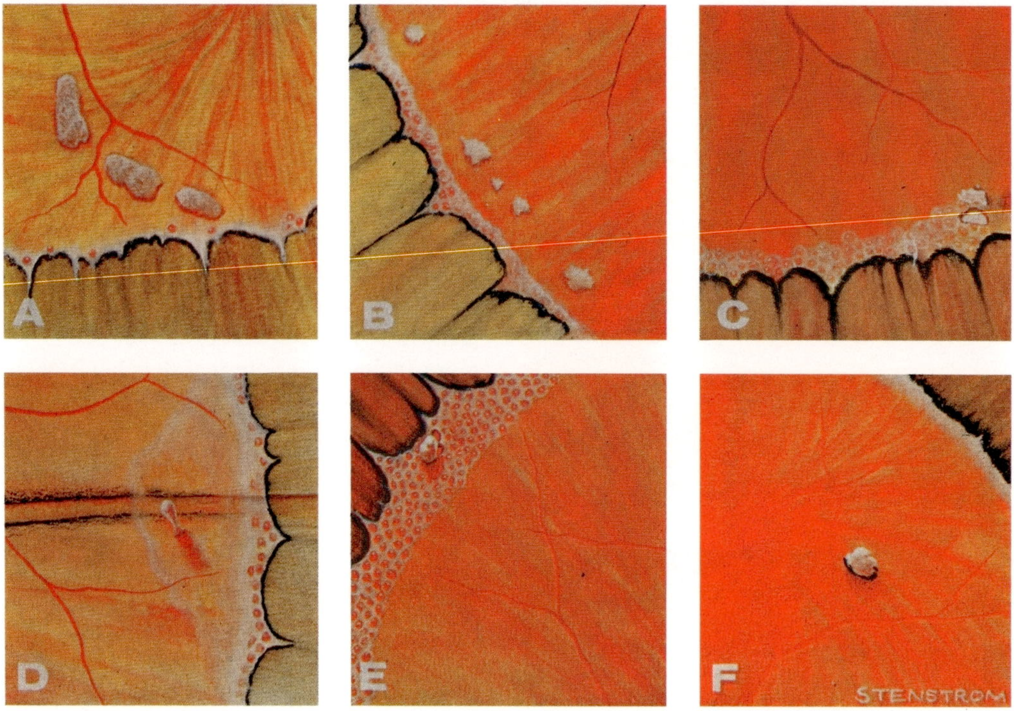

Figure 3-13 *Granular tissue in periphery of normal fundi. (A) Three granular patches in inferior periphery. (B) Five granular patches in nasal periphery. (C) Granular patch in inferior fundus periphery was torn off retina, causing incomplete retinal tear; tiny tag was partly torn from retina, causing small incomplete tear. (D) Nasal periphery with granular globule. Near long ciliary nerve, in area of white with pressure. (E) Nasal periphery with marked cystoid degeneration; granular globule was partly torn from retina, causing two incomplete retinal tears. (F) Temporal periphery with granular globule surrounded by fine line of pigment. All paintings in Figures 3-10 and 3-13 are exact reproductions of individual fundi.*

Reproduced from Rutnin U, Schepens CL: Fundus appearance in normal eyes. Am J Ophthalmol *1967; 64:821–852, 1040–1078. Published with permission from The American Journal of Ophthalmology. Copyright by The Ophthalmic Publishing Company.*

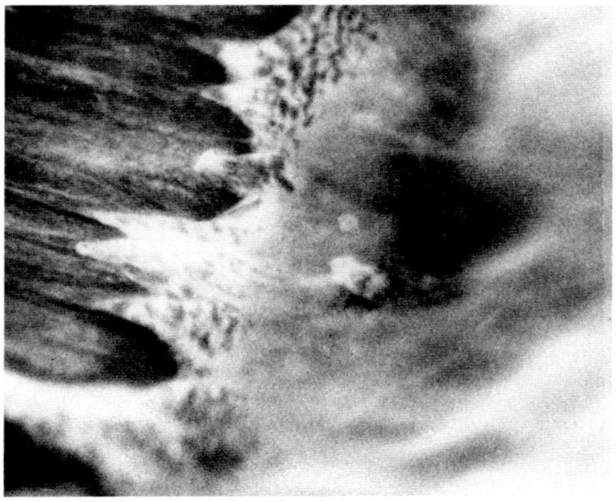

Figure 3-14 *Autopsy photograph of cystic retinal tuft. Reproduced with permission from Spencer LM, Straatsma BR, Foos RY: Tractional degenerations of the peripheral retina. In:* Symposium on Retina and Retinal Surgery *(Transactions of the New Orleans Academy of Ophthalmology). St Louis: CV Mosby Co; 1969:103–127.*

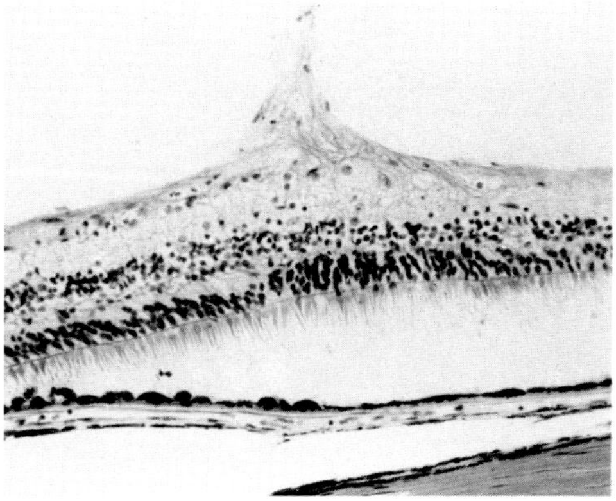

Figure 3-15 *Photomicrograph of retinal tuft. Reproduced with permission from Spencer LM, Straatsma BR, Foos RY: Tractional degenerations of the peripheral retina. In:* Symposium on Retina and Retinal Surgery *(Transactions of the New Orleans Academy of Ophthalmology). St Louis: CV Mosby Co; 1969:103–127.*

ment granules migrate into a pattern that looks like a fishnet or honeycomb (Figure 3-16; see also Figure 3-12C). The course of the degeneration is benign.

3-12-3 Equatorial Drusen

Drusen are more common in the equator than in the macula. Equatorial drusen may be associated with reticular pigmentary degeneration and are most often found in the elderly. They usually occur in the nasal periphery and are either punctate or geographic (see Figure 3-12D).

3-12-4 Paving-Stone Degeneration

Also known as *cobblestone degeneration* or *peripheral chorioretinal atrophy*, paving-stone degeneration is frequently found in the fundus periphery, usually in the inferior periphery (Figures 3-17, 3-18; see also

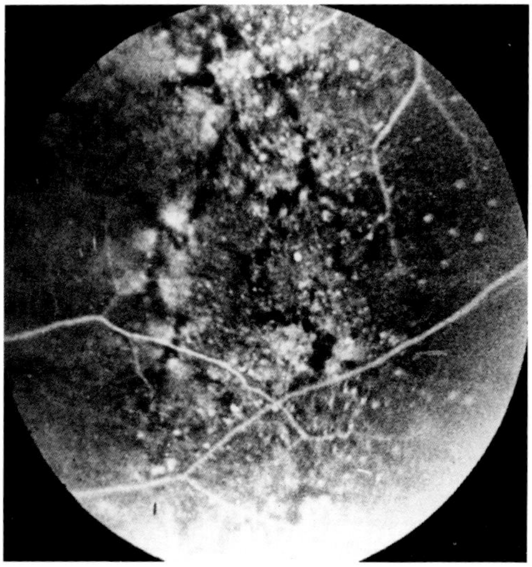

Figure 3-16 *Fluorescein angiogram of reticular pigmentary degeneration.*

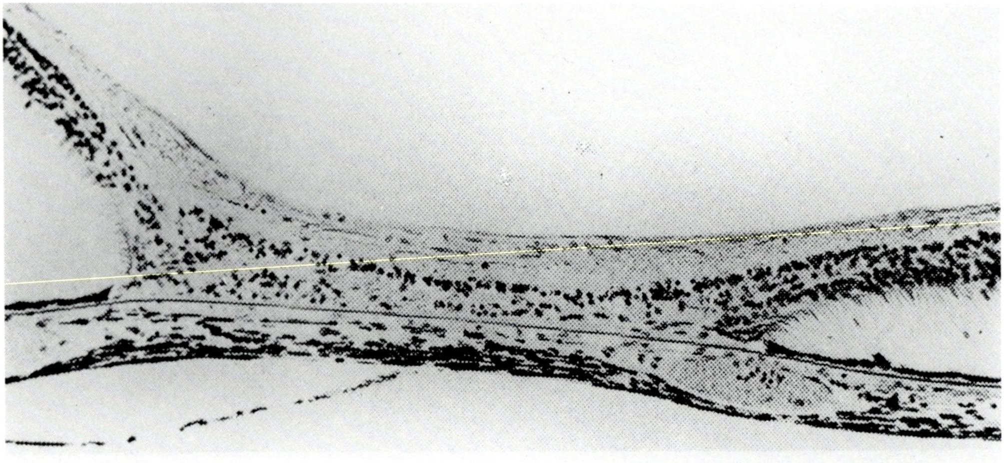

Figure 3-17 *Photomicrograph of paving-stone degeneration.*

Reproduced with permission from O'Malley P, Allen RA, Straatsma BR, O'Malley CC: Paving-stone degeneration of the retina. Arch Ophthalmol *1965;73: 169–182. Copyright 1965 American Medical Association.*

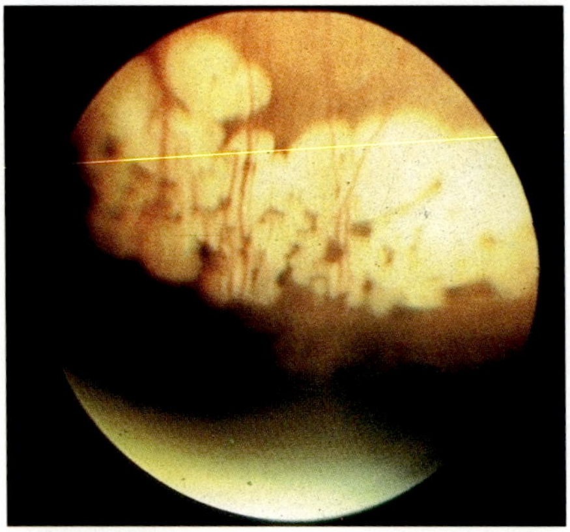

Figure 3-18 *Fundus photograph of confluent paving-stone lesions.*

Figure 3-12E). These lesions consist of circumscribed areas of atrophy in which there is loss of the outer layers of the retina, retinal pigment epithelium, choriocapillaris, and most of the choroidal vessels. Therefore, in an ophthalmoscopic examination of these lesions, the white sclera is revealed, with perhaps a few intact choroidal vessels crossing the defect. Clumps of pigment may be noted at the margin of each lesion.

An isolated lesion is 1 or 2 disc diameters in size, but adjacent lesions may coalesce to form an elongated lesion with a scalloped margin parallel to the ora. Sometimes the posterior edge of a large area of confluent paving stones creates the impression of a serrated dividing line and consequently has been called a *pseudo-ora* (see Figure 3-18). Rare secondary retinal breaks at the site of paving-stone lesions have been reported, but this form of degeneration is not a significant cause of primary retinal breaks.

3-12-5 Retinal Whitening

A common condition, whitening of the retina is ordinarily apparent without pressure from the scleral indentor, and this fact is referred to by the notation "white without pressure." But if it is evident only when pressure is applied, it is described as "white with pressure." Areas of peripheral whitening sometimes assume rather bizarre forms with geographic outlines, and they are not always connected with the ora serrata. Generally, the areas of whiteness are anterior to the equator, but occasionally they extend to the posterior pole. When examined with scleral indentation, they are discovered to be flat, which differentiates them from retinal detachment or retinoschisis (see Figure 3-12F). Infrequently, a round area of normal fundus is surrounded by whitening, creating the incorrect impression of a retinal hole surrounded by a flat retinal detachment.

Whitening is assumed to result from alterations in the anatomy of the vitreoretinal interface. It is more marked in pigmented races and is virtually universal among blacks.

3-12-6 Pars Plana Cysts

Pars plana cysts are relatively common (Figure 3-19; see Figure 3-12G). They average from 1 to 3 disc diameters in size and appear transparent. Scleral indentation clearly reveals their elevation. Pars plana cysts are usually multiple, bilateral, located temporally, and limited to the posterior half of the pars plana. They are clinically benign and do not evolve into retinoschisis.

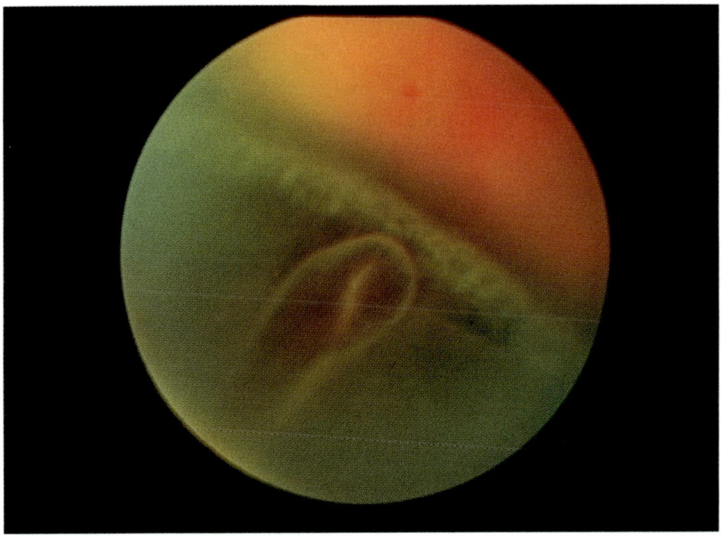

Figure 3-19 *Fundus photograph of pars plana cyst.*
Courtesy Norman E. Byer, MD.

3-12-7 Retinal Erosion

Isolated areas of loss of substance in the inner retinal layers are referred to as *retinal erosion*. These focal lesions are curiosities and do not predispose to retinal detachment (see Figure 3-12H).

3-12-8 Pigment Clumps

Small pigment clumps frequently noted in the peripheral fundus are generally insignificant. Occasionally, however, a vitreoretinal adhesion associated with pigment clumps does appear, and this adhesion may produce a retinal tear. The prognosis for pigment clumps without tears is good, and prophylactic therapy is not indicated.

3-13

DIAGNOSIS OF RETINAL DETACHMENT

An obvious detachment is recognizable by the marked elevation of the retina. The retina appears opaque, its blood vessels are relatively dark, it may lie in folds, and the detached retina may undulate. A shallow, slightly elevated detachment of the retina can be more difficult to diagnose. Stereopsis afforded by the binocular indirect ophthalmoscope enhances recognition and proper evaluation of the characteristics unique to each detachment. It is helpful to examine the normal attached retina, then compare with the adjacent area in question for any changes in retinal transparency that may suggest detachment. With fundus biomicroscopy, a shadow of the retinal vessels is cast on the pigment epithelium. A small degree of shadow formation may be found in the normal retina, but prominent separation between the retinal vessel and its underlying shadow is the clue to a shallow detachment. The detached retina may assume an "orange-peel appearance," which is best seen when the retina is viewed in light reflected from the choroid. If a shallow detachment in the periphery is suspected, scleral indentation usually enables visualization of the subtle retinal separation.

The limits of the retinal detachment should be recorded on the fundus chart. In the search for retinal breaks, the distribution of fluid is a valuable clue to the loation of the break(s). It should not be assumed that the detachment is limited by the ora serrata, and a careful search for detachment of the pars plana is required. The limit of the detachment may be accentuated by the presence of a demarcation line, either pigmented or nonpigmented (Figure 3-20).

Elevation of the retinal surface can represent a retinal detachment, but elevation can also be caused by retinoschisis, that is, splitting within the sensory retina. When retinoschisis accompanies detachment, it always predates the onset of detachment (see Figure 6-28). An attempt should be made to record the extent of the schisis cavity, as well as the area of detached retina. But this is often difficult, and sometimes the extent is not clear until the characteristic appearance of retinoschisis becomes better defined during cryotherapy. A diagnostic feature of retinoschisis is the "white Swiss cheese" appearance of the outer layer of the schistic retina as it is frozen, in contrast to the dull orange change that occurs at the level of the retinal pigment epithelium, deep to the overlying detached retina, when viewed during cryotherapy.

Intraretinal macrocysts, which are defined as focal secondary retinoschisis, may mimic degenerative retinoschisis. They occur only in long-standing detachments. Intraretinal macrocysts are usually 2 or 3 disc diameters in size and are most often found in the periphery. Macrocysts require no special treatment and disappear after retinal reattachment.

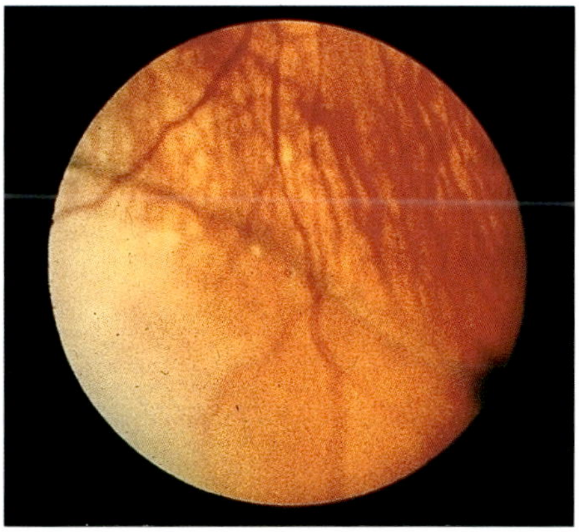

Figure 3-20 *Fundus photograph of subtle demarcation line.*

3-14

DETECTION OF RETINAL BREAKS

The entire retina should be carefully examined for retinal breaks by binocular indirect ophthalmoscopy, supplemented by scleral indentation for the periphery. While breaks may be found in any area, the distribution of the subretinal fluid is a clue to the most likely location of a primary retinal break (Figure 3-21). If one superior quadrant is detached, the break is apt to be near the upper edge of the detachment. When the superior half of the retina is detached, the break is most likely near the 12-o'clock meridian. An inferior quadrantic detachment usually has the break near the upper edge of the detachment or in the meridian bisecting the area of detachment. If the inferior half is detached, the break is probably near the 6-o'clock meridian. However, when the

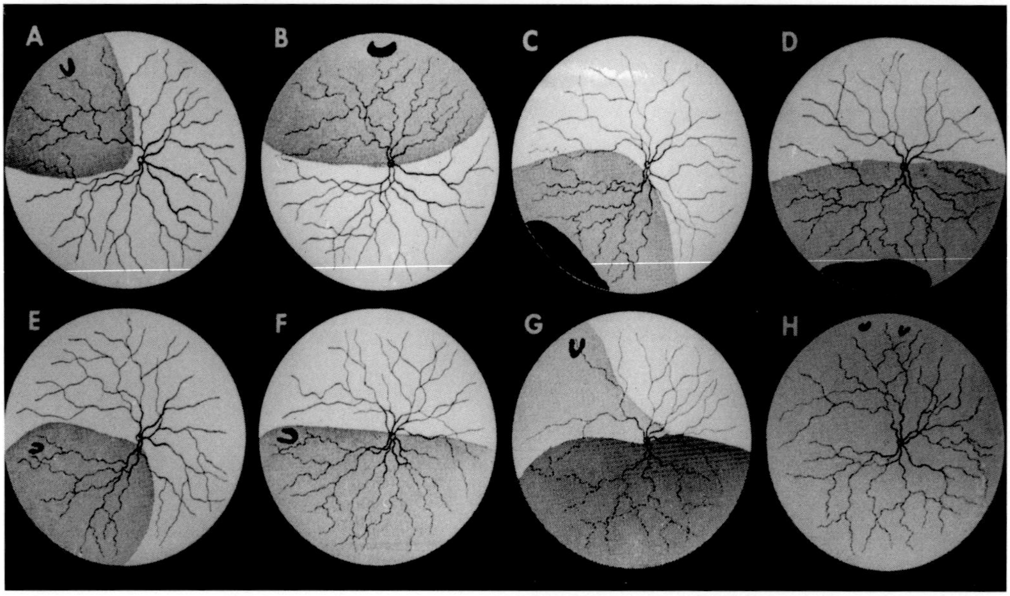

Figure 3-21 *Most probable site of retinal break as suggested by distribution of subretinal fluid.* *Courtesy Charles L. Schepens, MD.*

fluid is higher on one side of an inferior detachment than on the other, the break is usually on the higher side. In total retinal detachment, the break is almost always between the 10- and 2-o'clock meridians. If there are inferior bullae, the examiner should assume that a retinal break is above the horizontal meridian. In the presence of a demarcation line, the break is often found in the meridian that bisects the demarcated area (Figure 3-22).

The history may provide a clue to the location of a break. When the detachment has progressed rapidly, the break is usually superior, fairly large, and probably located nearer the equator than the ora. If the history suggests slow progression of the detachment, a small, inferior, or extremely peripheral break should be sought. The quadrant of first detectable field loss is a valuable indication of the lo-

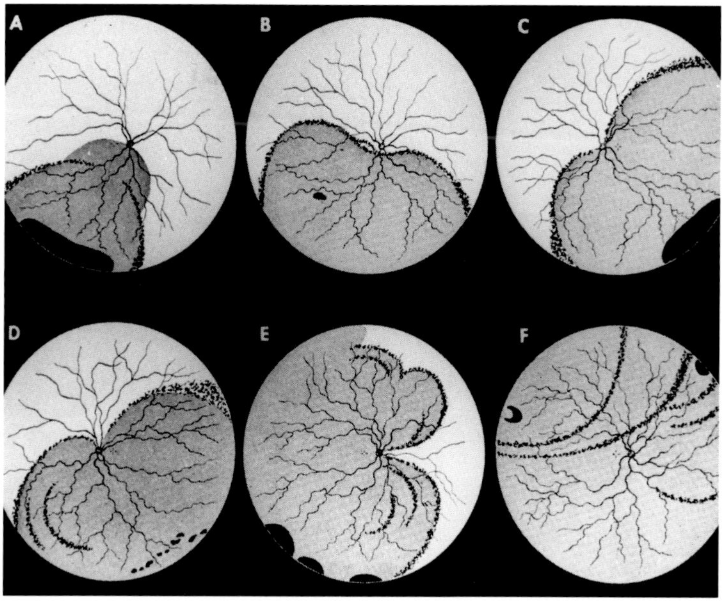

Figure 3-22 *Probable site of retinal break as suggested by orientation of demarcation lines.*

Courtesy Charles L. Schepens, MD.

cation of the primary break, particularly if the detachment has become total. Special attention should be paid to all areas of abnormality, particularly lattice degeneration, meridional folds, pigmentation, opercula, and hemorrhage.

A red lesion may be either a retinal hole or a retinal hemorrhage. Careful examination will reveal a homogeneous red color for retinal hemorrhage, somewhat denser than the reddish choroid seen through a retinal break. Most importantly, while both lesions are similar in color, hemorrhage has a solid appearance compared to the translucent quality of a retinal void. Parallax in ophthalmoscopy is helpful, because retinal hemorrhage is localized in the plane of the retina, whereas the apparent redness of a hole is in the plane of the pigment epithelium. The most valuable technique for differentiation is scleral indentation, which shows whether there is retinal hemorrhage or a break in the plane of the retina.

3-15

EVALUATION OF THE MACULA

If the macula has not yet been detached, a judgment should be made about the imminence of this serious event. The threat of extension into the macula is relatively high if the break is superotemporal or equatorial instead of at the ora. The threat of immediate involvement of the macula by the retinal detachment is relatively low if the break is inferior, on the nasal side, or near the ora serrata.

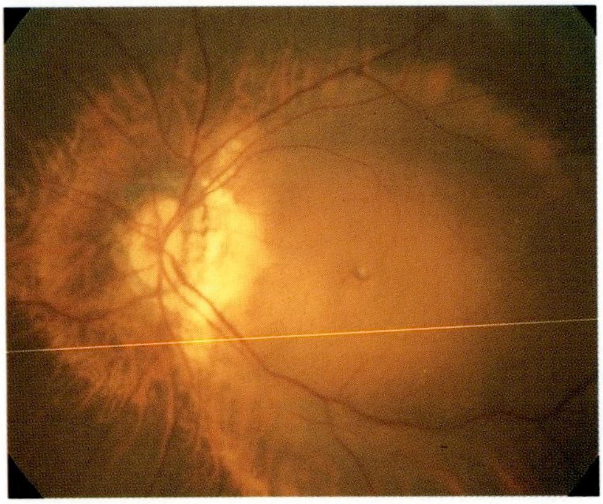

Figure 3-23 *Retinal detachment caused by macular break in high myopia.*
Courtesy C. P. Wilkinson, MD.

Normal visual acuity rules out detachment of the macula, but poor vision is not a definitive indication. Poor vision may also be due to antecedent macular or optic nerve disease, amblyopia, or opacities of the media. Subtle degrees of macular detachment are best evaluated stereoscopically with the slit lamp and contact lens. The luteal pigment of the macula, xanthophyll, is not readily apparent in the normal macula, but becomes more evident as a yellow color against the background of intraretinal edema when detachment includes the macula.

Apparent holes in the macula are relatively common in retinal detachment, but true macular holes are rare. Macular breaks as a cause of retinal detachment are usually seen in association with the staphyloma of high myopia or following trauma (Figure 3-23).

3-16

PROLIFERATIVE VITREORETINOPATHY

The most common cause of failure in retinal surgery is the presence of intravitreal, preretinal, or subretinal membranes. The various gradations of proliferative vitreoretinopathy (PVR), as published by the Retina Society Terminology Committee in 1983 (see Suggested Readings), are summarized in Table 3-3 and Figure 3-24. An updated classification, published by Machemer and associates in 1991 (see Suggested Readings), offers several advantages, including recognition of *anterior* PVR (Tables 3-4 and 3-5). The 1991 classification has been used in several research publications, but most clinical papers continue to employ the 1983 classification.

TABLE 3-3

Classification of Retinal Detachment With Proliferative Vitreoretinopathy, 1983

Grade	Name	Clinical Signs
A	Minimal	Vitreous haze, vitreous pigment clumps
B	Moderate	Wrinkling of inner retinal surface, rolled edge of retinal break, retinal stiffness, vessel tortuosity
C	Marked	Full-thickness fixed retinal folds
		C-1 One quadrant
		C-2 Two quadrants
		C-3 Three quadrants
D	Massive	Fixed retinal folds in four quadrants
		D-1 Wide funnel shape
		D-2 Narrow funnel shape*
		D-3 Closed funnel (optic nerve head not visible)

**Existence of narrow funnel shape is evidenced by indirect ophthalmoscopy when anterior end of funnel can be seen within 45° field of +20 D condensing lens (Nikon or equivalent).*

Source: Retina Society Terminology Committee: The classification of retinal detachment with proliferative vitreoretinopathy. Ophthalmology *1983;90:121–125. See also Machemer et al, in Suggested Readings.*

TABLE 3-4

Classification of Proliferative Vitreoretinopathy, 1991

Grade	Features
A	Vitreous haze, vitreous pigment clumps, pigment clusters on inferior retina
B	Wrinkling of inner retinal surface, retinal stiffness, vessel tortuosity, rolled and irregular edge of retinal break, decreased mobility of vitreous
C P 1–12	Posterior to equator: focal, diffuse, or circumferential full-thickness folds,* subretinal strands*
C A 1–12	Anterior to equator: focal, diffuse, or circumferential full-thickness folds,* subretinal strands,* anterior displacement,* condensed vitreous with strands

**Expressed in number of clock hours involved.*

Source: Machemer R, Aaberg TM, Freeman HM, et al: An updated classification of retinal detachment with proliferative vitreoretinopathy. Am J Ophthalmol *1991; 112:159–165. Published with permission from The American Journal of Ophthalmology. Copyright by The Ophthalmic Publishing Company.*

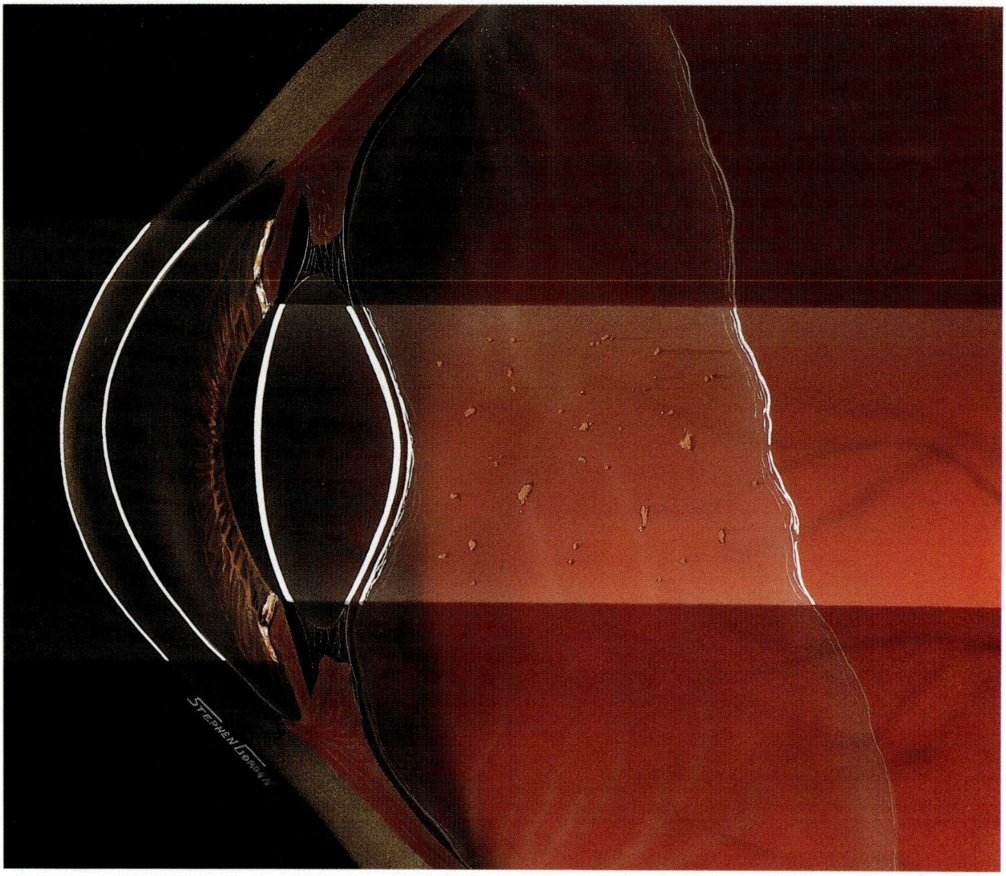

A

Figure 3-24 *Proliferative vitreoretinopathy (PVR). (A) Grade A, pigment clumps. (B) Grade B, surface wrinkling in 7:30-o'clock meridian. (C) Grade B, rolled-over posterior edge of retinal break.*

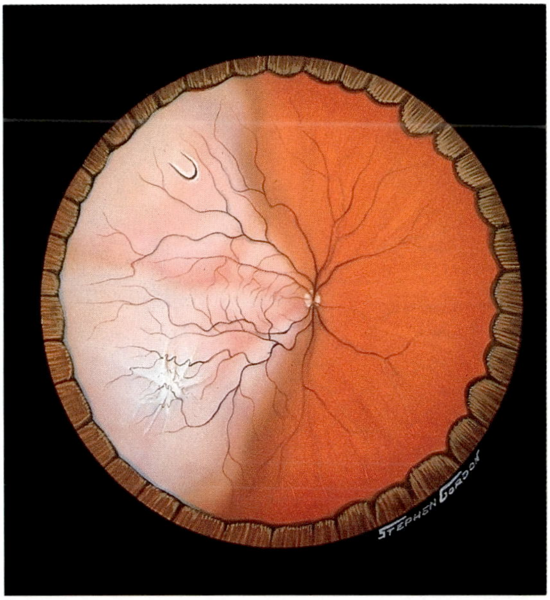

B

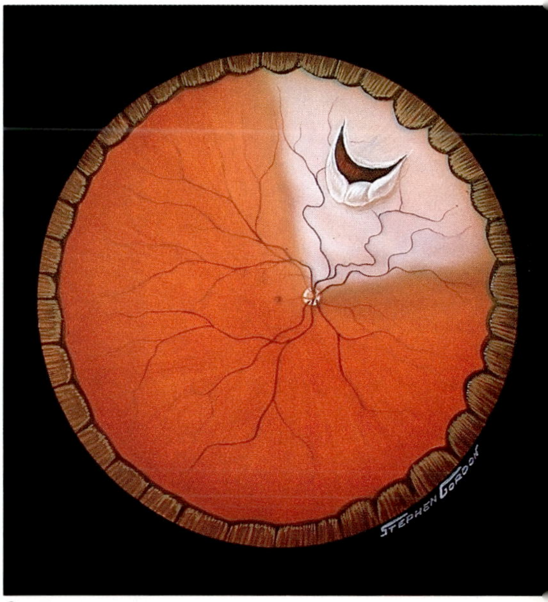

C

TABLE 3-5

Grade C Proliferative Vitreoretinopathy Described by Contraction Type, 1991

Type	Location in Relation to Equator	Features
Focal	Posterior	Starfold posterior to vitreous base
Diffuse	Posterior	Confluent starfolds posterior to vitreous base; optic disc may not be visible
Subretinal	Posterior/ anterior	Proliferations under retina: annular strand near disc, linear strands, moth-eaten–appearing sheets
Circumferential	Anterior	Contraction along posterior edge of vitreous base with central displacement of retina, peripheral retina stretched, posterior retina in radial folds
Anterior displacement	Anterior	Vitreous base pulled anteriorly by proliferative tissue, peripheral retinal trough, ciliary processes may be stretched and may be covered by membrane, iris may be retracted

Source: Machemer R, Aaberg TM, Freeman HM, et al: An updated classification of retinal detachment with proliferative vitreoretinopathy. Am J Ophthalmol *1991; 112:159–165. Published with permission from The American Journal of Ophthalmology. Copyright by The Ophthalmic Publishing Company.*

Figure 3-24 *(D) Grade C-1, one quadrant of full-thickness retinal folds. (E) Grade C-2, two quadrants of full-thickness retinal folds.*

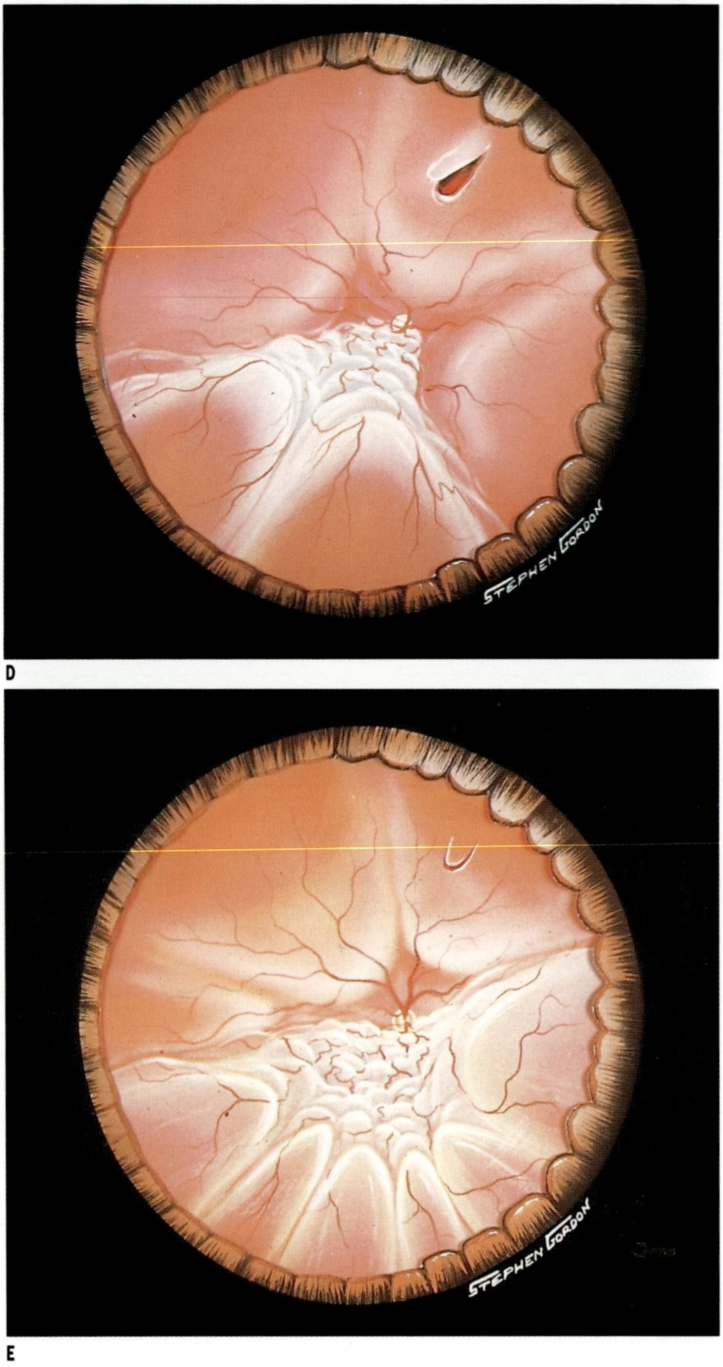

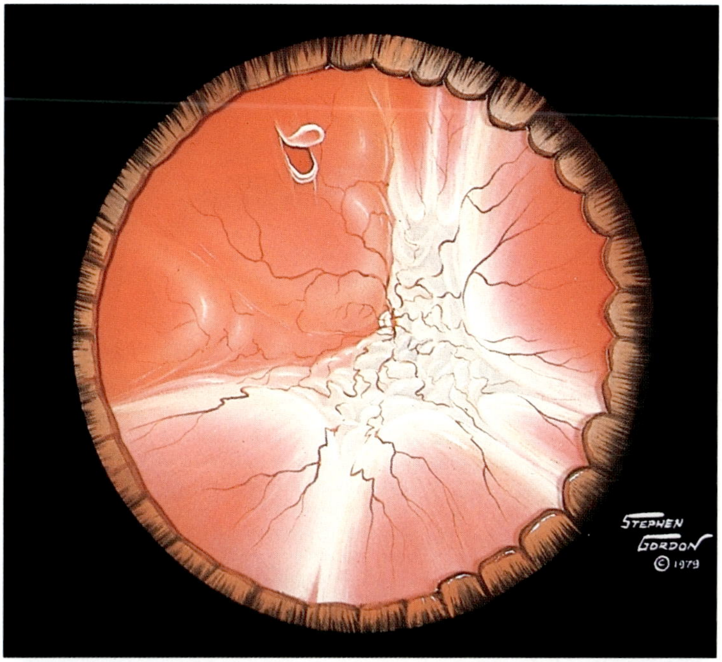

F

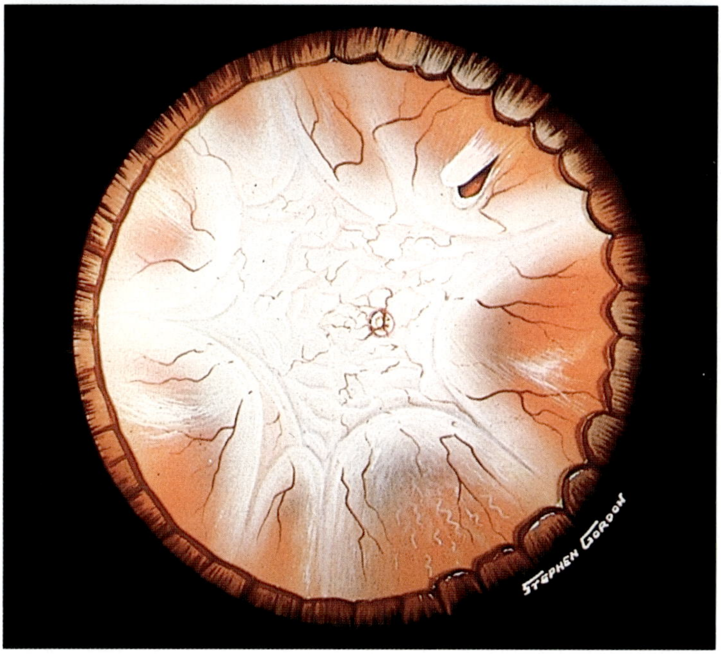

G

Figure 3-24 *(F) Grade C-3, three quadrants of full-thickness retinal folds. (G) Grade D-1, four quadrants of full-thickness retinal folds with wide retinal funnel configuration.*

Figure 3-24 *(H) Grade D-1, wide retinal funnel configuration. (I) Grade D-2, narrow retinal funnel configuration.*

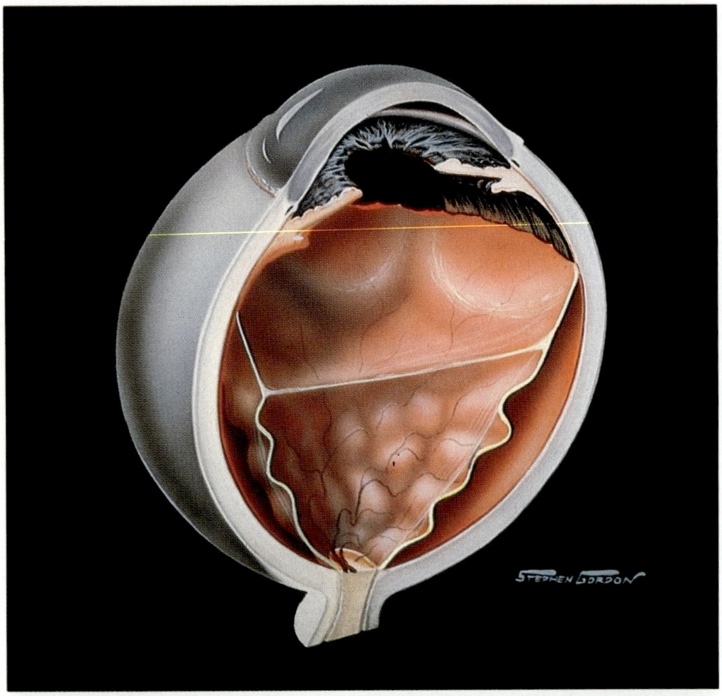

H

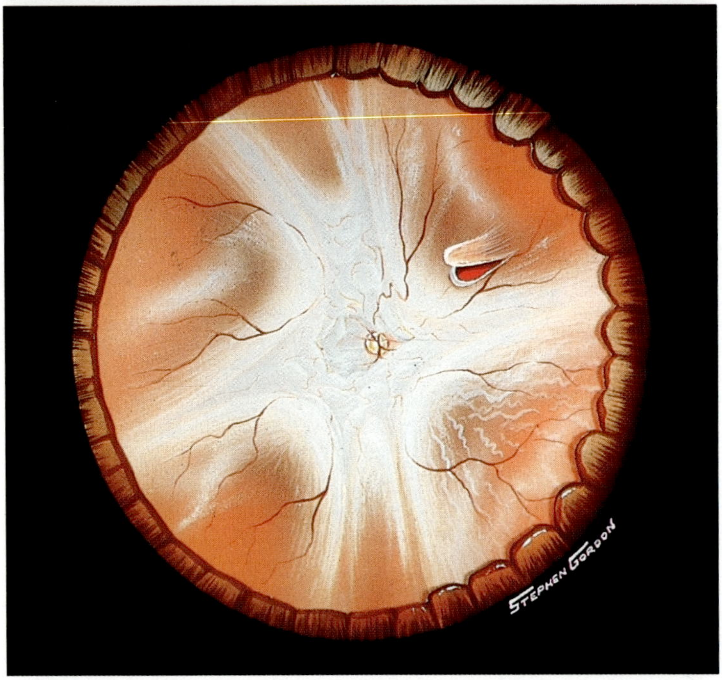

I

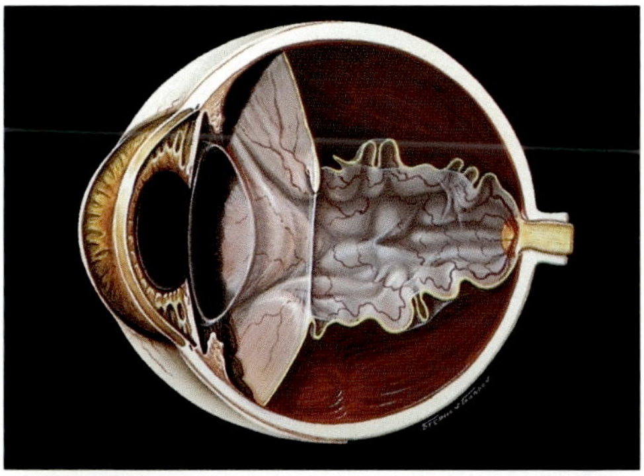

J

Figure 3-24 *(J) Grade D-2, narrow retinal funnel configuration. (K) If anterior entrance to retinal funnel can be visualized within 45° field of +20 D indirect ophthalmoscope lens (Nikon or equivalent), funnel is designated as "narrow."*

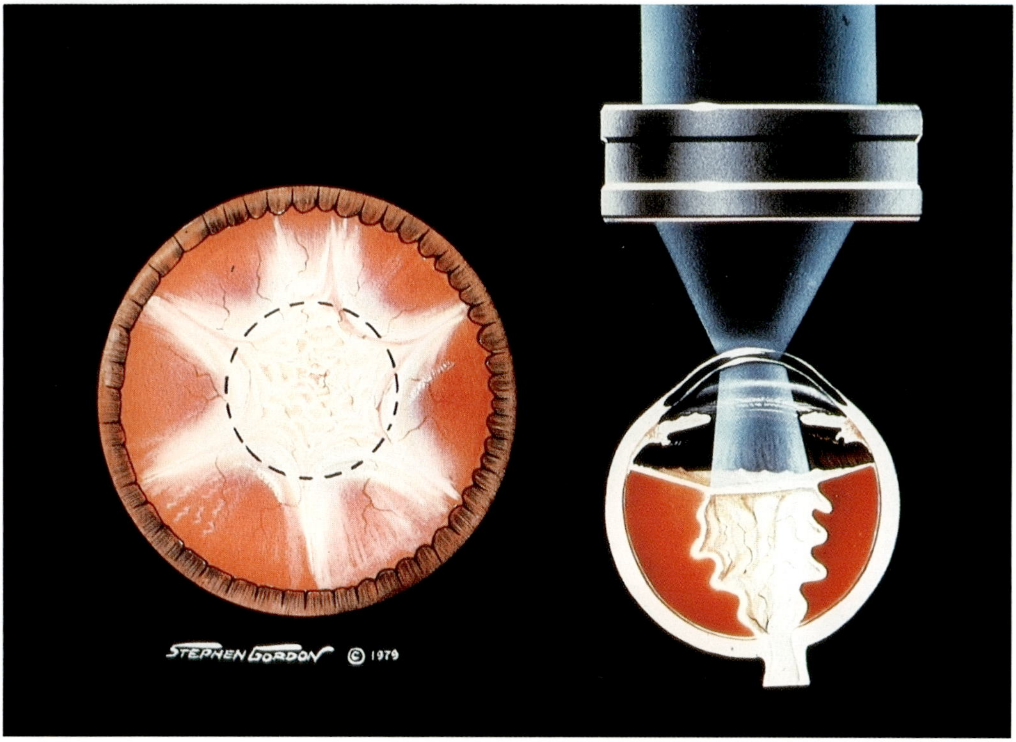

K

Figure 3-24 *(L) Grade D-3, closed funnel, obscuring view of optic nerve head. (M) Grade D-3, closed funnel, obscuring view of optic nerve head.*

Reproduced with permission from Retina Society Terminology Committee: The classification of retinal detachment with proliferative vitreoretinopathy. Ophthalmology *1983: 90:121–125.*

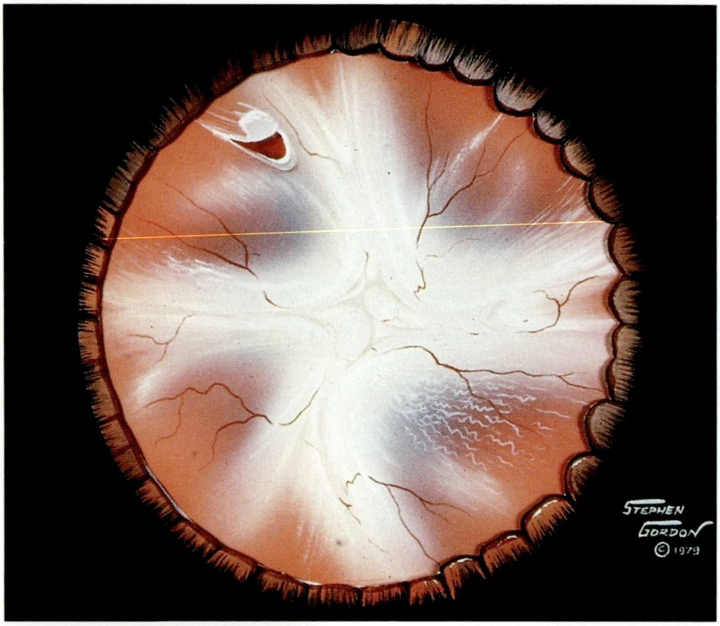

L

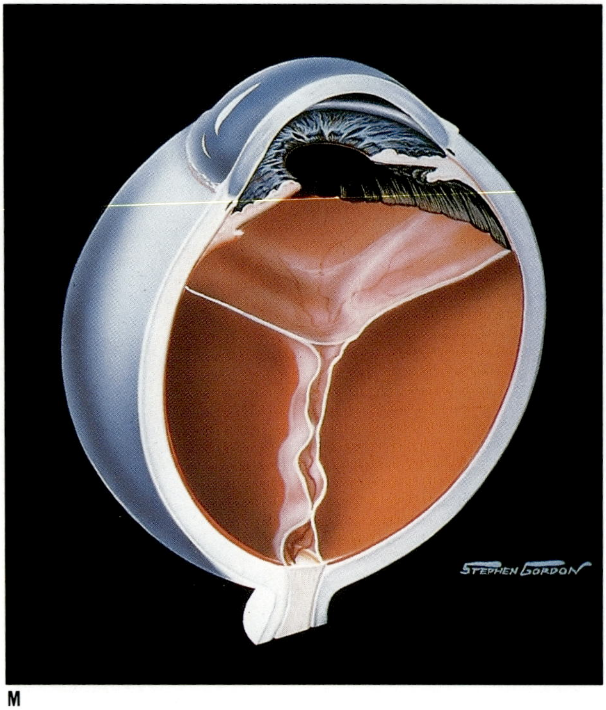

M

Far-advanced PVR is recognized by whitening of the retina, which is drawn in toward the visual axis with numerous fixed folds centered about the optic disc. The presence of a preretinal membrane can be subtle and may not be directly observed, but its presence can be inferred from the finding of fixed retinal folds—folds that do not undulate with eye movement. These folds may be circumferential or meridional. The most diagnostic of these is the star fold. Posterior rolling of the posterior edge of the retinal break is another sign of preretinal organization.

Some long-standing detachments develop subretinal fibrosis. This is clinically recognized by linear, curved, and angular yellow-white lines on the retroretinal surface of the detached retina (Figure 3-25).

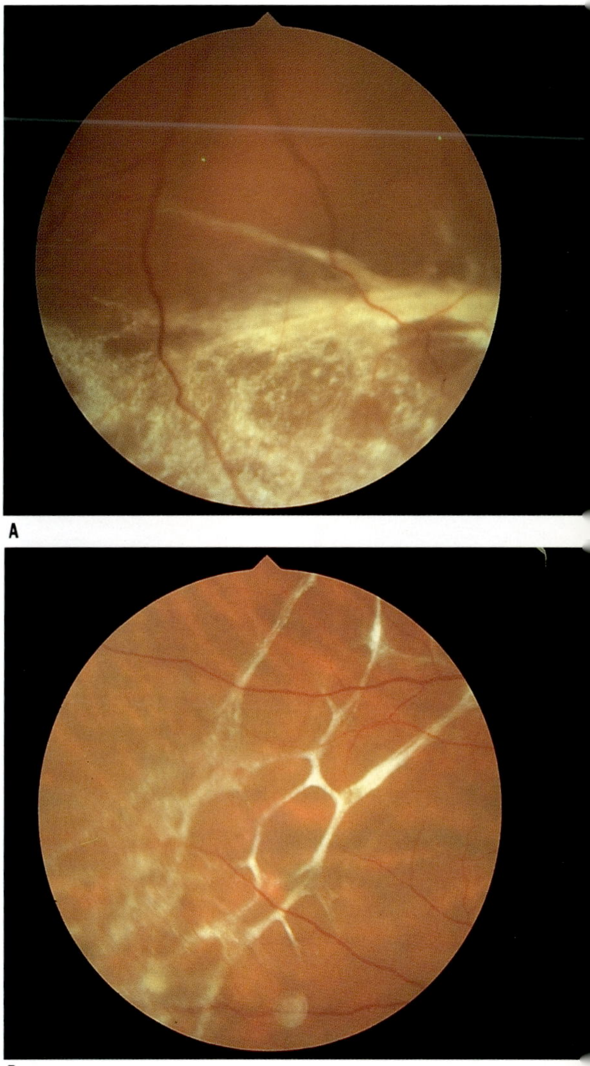

A

B

Figure 3-25 *Fundus photographs of subretinal fibrosis. (A) Diffuse sheet with strands. (B) Multiple strands.*

Courtesy Elaine L. Chuang, MD.

3-17

DIFFERENTIAL DIAGNOSIS

Rhegmatogenous retinal detachments must be differentiated from exudative and tractional detachments. More than 90% of all clinical detachments are of the rhegmatogenous type. The diagnostic features of all three types are summarized in Table 3-6. Various lesions that may simulate retinal detachment must also be carefully identified. The four most common lesions that are confused with rhegmatogenous retinal detachment are malignant melanoma of the choroid with associated detachment, inflammatory detachment, choroidal detachment, and degenerative retinoschisis. The differential diagnosis of nonrhegmatogenous retinal detachment and lesions that simulate detachment is summarized in Table 3-7.

TABLE 3-6

Diagnostic Features of the Three Types of Retinal Detachments

	Rhegmatogenous (Primary)	Nonrhegmatogenous (Secondary)	
		Exudative	*Tractional*
History	Aphakia, myopia, blunt trauma, photopsia, floaters, field defect; generally healthy	Systemic factors such as malignant hypertension, eclampsia, renal failure	Diabetes, prematurity, penetrating trauma, sickle cell disease
Retinal break	Identified in 90% to 95% of cases	No break, or coincidental	No primary break; may develop secondary break
Extent of detachment	Extends to ora early	Gravity-dependent; extension to ora is variable	Frequently does not extend to ora
Retinal mobility	Undulating bullae or folds	Smoothly elevated bullae, usually without folds	Taut retina, concave surface, peaks to traction points
Retinal elevation	Low to moderate, seldom extreme	Varies—may be extremely high to approximate lens	Elevated to level of focal traction
Evidence of chronicity	Demarcation lines, intraretinal macrocysts, atrophic retina	Usually none	Demarcation lines
Pigment in vitreous	Present in 70% of cases	Not present	Present in trauma cases
Vitreous changes	Frequently syneretic, posterior vitreous detachment, traction on flap of tear	Usually clear, except in uveitis	Vitreoretinal traction
Subretinal fluid	Clear	May be turbid and shift rapidly to dependent location with changes in head position	Clear, no shift
Choroidal mass	None	May be present	None
Intraocular pressure	Frequently low	Varies	Usually normal
Transillumination	Normal	Blocked transillumination if pigmented choroidal lesion present	Normal
Examples of conditions causing detachment	Retinal break	Uveitis, metastatic tumor, malignant melanoma, angiomatosis, Coats' disease, Eale's disease, Harada's syndrome, retinoblastoma, choroidal hemangioma, senile exudative maculopathy, optic pit, exudative detachment after cryotherapy or diathermy	Proliferative diabetic retinopathy, retinopathy of prematurity, toxocara, sickle cell retinopathy, posttraumatic vitreous traction

TABLE 3-7

Differential Diagnosis of Nonrhegmatogenous Retinal Detachment and Lesions That Simulate Detachment

Nonrhegmatogenous Detachment	Lesions Simulating Detachment
Exudative	*Vitreal*
Primary tumors	Membranes
Malignant melanoma of choroid	Hemorrhage
Hemangioma of choroid	Inflammation
Retinoblastoma	*Retinal*
Metastic tumors to choroid, especially from breast or lung	Primary retinoschisis
Inflammation	Juvenile
Scleritis	Degenerative
Choroiditis, eg, Harada's disease	Secondary retinoschisis
Retinitis, eg, toxoplasmosis	Proliferative diabetic retinopathy
Vascular disease	Pars planitis
Angiomatosis of retina (von Hippel's disease)	Choroidal detachment
Telangiectasia retinae (juvenile and adult Coats' disease)	Serous
Eale's disease	Hemorrhage
Retinal vein occlusion	
Optic nerve disease	
Pit of optic nerve head with serous detachment of macula	
Nerve head drusen with serosanguineous detachment of adjacent retina	
Macular disease	
Central serous chorioretinopathy (can extend to ora serrata, rarely)	
Age-related macular degeneration	
Other causes of disciform detachment (eg, presumed ocular histoplasmosis, angioid streaks, high myopia)	
Systemic disease	
Toxemia	
Uremia	
Lupus erythematosus	
Leukemia	
Tractional	
Retinopathy of prematurity	
Sickle cell retinopathy	
Proliferative diabetic retinopathy	
Posttraumatic vitreous membranes	

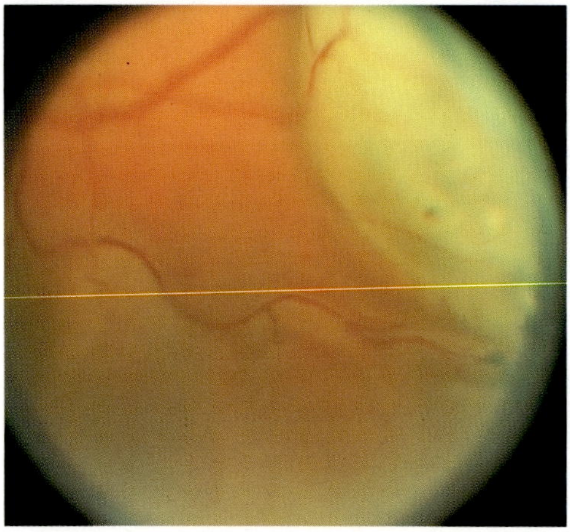

Figure 3-26 *Retinal detachment associated with malignant melanoma.*
Courtesy Devron R. Char, MD.

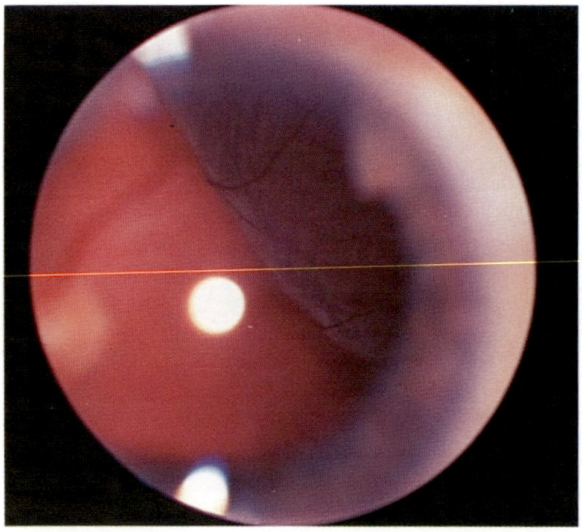

Figure 3-27 *Retina elevated by choroidal detachment.*
Reprinted with permission of Medcom, Inc., from Conor O'Malley, MD, FACS, and Patrick O'Malley, MD, FACS: "The Peripheral Fundus of the Eye."

Detachments associated with malignant melanoma are usually readily identified by visualizing the choroidal tumor with binocular indirect ophthalmoscopy (Figure 3-26), and the subretinal fluid usually shifts with changes in position of the head. "Shifting fluid" is defined as a *changing* of the detachment *borders* in response to changes in head position; it does not mean movement of the fluid within stable detachment borders. Shifting fluid is common in exudative detachments and in rare instances is also seen in old rhegmatogenous detachments.

Other techniques can also be employed to determine whether a tumor is present. With scleral transillumination, a pigmented tumor blocks light. Fluorescein angiography typically shows subretinal hyperfluorescence of a tumor. If the media are not clear, a tumor can be demonstrated by ultrasonography.

An inflammatory detachment is characterized by a transparent retina with an unusually clear view of the underlying choroid. Signs of inflammation with flare and cells are seen during slit-lamp examination of the vitreous, and inflammatory lesions of the choroid can usually be seen with indirect ophthalmoscopy. Retinitis is manifested by a fluffy white retinal lesion with turbidity of the vitreous.

Choroidal detachment is usually bullous, and nasal or temporal bullae tend to be larger than superior and inferior bullae (Figure 3-27). Usually, the brown choroid can be seen immediately beneath the retina. In the deep valleys between choroidal bullae, the choroid is tethered to the sclera by the vortex veins or along the course of the long posterior ciliary artery and nerve. This tethering effect tends to limit the posterior extension of the detachment, and therefore the posterior pole is often spared. There may be folds in the posterior pole but no frank detachment. While retinal detachment usually extends anteriorly only as far as the ora serrata, detachment of the choroid extends anteriorly to the scleral spur. Most choroidal detachments are serous, but occasionally a hemorrhagic detachment is seen. Serous and hemorrhagic detachments can be readily differentiated by scleral transillumination. There are many causes for choroidal detachment, but the most common is hypotony following intraocular surgery, especially surgery for cataract.

The differential diagnosis of retinal detachment must also include retinoschisis, as discussed in Chapter 2.

SUGGESTED READINGS

Brockhurst RJ: Nanophthalmos with uveal effusion: a new clinical entity. *Arch Ophthalmol* 1975;93:1989–1999.

Burton TC, Arafat NL, Phelps CD: Intraocular pressure in retinal detachment. *Int Ophthalmol* 1979;1:147–152.

Dobbie JG, Phillips CI: Detachment of ora serrata and pars ciliaris retinae in "idiopathic" retinal detachment. *Arch Ophthalmol* 1962; 168:610–614.

Gass JDM: Bullous retinal detachment: an unusual manifestation of idiopathic central serous choroidopathy. *Am J Ophthalmol* 1973;75: 810–821.

Gass JD, Jallow S: Idiopathic serous detachment of the choroid, ciliary body, and retina (uveal effusion syndrome). *Ophthalmology* 1982;89:1018–1032.

Griffith RD, Ryan EA, Hilton GF: Primary retinal detachments without apparent breaks. *Am J Ophthalmol* 1976;81:420–427.

Grignolo A, Schepens CL, Heath P: Cysts of the pars plana ciliaris. *Arch Ophthalmol* 1957; 58:530–543.

Gutman FA, Zegarra H: Retinal detachment secondary to retinal branch vein occlusion. *Trans Am Acad Ophthalmol Otolaryngol* 1976; 81:491–496.

Hagler WS, North AW: Intraretinal macrocysts and retinal detachment. *Trans Am Acad Ophthalmol Otolaryngol* 1967;71:442–454.

Machemer R, Aaberg TM, Freeman HM, et al: An updated classification of retinal detachment with proliferative vitreoretinopathy. *Am J Ophthalmol* 1991;112:159–165.

Marcus DF, Aaberg TM: Intraretinal macrocysts in retinal detachment. *Arch Ophthalmol* 1979;97:1273–1275.

Phelps CD, Burton TC: Glaucoma and retinal detachment. *Arch Ophthalmol* 1977;95:418–422.

Retinal Society Terminology Committee: The classification of retinal detachment with proliferative vitreoretinopathy. *Ophthalmology* 1983; 90:121–125.

Rubin ML: The optics of indirect ophthalmoscopy. *Surv Ophthalmol* 1964;9:449–464.

Rutnin U, Schepens CL: Fundus appearance in normal eyes. *Am J Ophthalmol* 1967;64: 821–852, 1040–1078.

Schepens CL: Diagnostic and prognostic factors as found in preoperative examination. *Trans Am Acad Ophthalmol Otolaryngol* 1952; 56:398–412.

Seelenfreund MH, Kraushar MF, Schepens CL, et al: Choroidal detachment associated with primary retinal detachment. *Arch Ophthalmol* 1974;91:254–258.

CHAPTER 4

Preoperative Management

Prior to surgery, the physician must counsel the patient, write appropriate preoperative orders, and manage existing complications. An informed patient is apt to be more cooperative and ultimately better reconciled to the therapeutic outcome.

4-1

PREOPERATIVE COUNSELING

The principal determinant of doctor–patient rapport is probably the manner in which the preoperative discussion is conducted. After the preoperative examination, the patient's family should be invited to join the discussion with the patient and physician. They should be informed of the diagnosis, and some comment should be made about the status of the other eye. Some basic information regarding the nature of retinal detachment will be greatly appreciated by both patient and family. The prognosis should be briefly described, the possibility of reoperation mentioned, and the probable visual outcome discussed. If the macula is not detached, the physician should explain that some patients (approximately 10%) will lose a few lines of visual acuity. If the macula is detached, the ophthalmologist should explain that retinal reattachment is not paralleled by functional recovery and that full visual recovery should not be expected. The patient should also be told of the probable length of hospitalization and convalescence.

Informed consent is both a medical and a legal requirement. The alternatives to surgery must be reviewed. The major complications of retinal detachment surgery should be mentioned; and if the patient indicates a desire for further details, such complications, including blindness, should be thoroughly discussed. The discussion should include some comment regarding possible systemic and anesthetic complications.

The financial commitment should be explained in detail. The patient should enter the hospital with a clear understanding of the fees for the surgeon, assistant surgeon, anesthesiologist, and internist as well as the charges for the hospital.

4-2

PREOPERATIVE ORDERS

Preoperative orders vary somewhat with each surgeon, but routine cases have been satisfactorily managed by one of the authors of this monograph (G.F.H.) with orders such as those that follow. These orders apply to a patient admitted the day of surgery for a general anesthetic procedure. However, scleral buckling can also be done as same-day surgery with local anesthesia for appropriate patients.

1. Complete blood count.

2. Electrocardiogram if patient is over 50 years old

3. Nothing by mouth (NPO) for 8 hours prior to surgery

4. Bathroom privileges

5. Inquiry regarding allergies and recording on front of chart

6. Notation of present medications

7. Scopolamine 0.25% and phenylephrine 2.5%; one drop of each in affected eye every 5 minutes, starting 45 minutes before surgery, for a total of three applications

8. Operative permit for ______________ of the _____ eye

9. Bedside box containing eight eye pads, 1-inch paper tape, and the postoperative instruction sheet

These routine orders should be modified as indicated for each case. A chest x-ray and additional laboratory tests should be ordered as needed. Many retinal surgeons prefer to have every patient examined preoperatively by an internist, but a surgeon may elect to obtain the history and perform the physical examination if the patient has no significant medical problems.

In certain instances, benefits are derived from the ocular rest resulting from bilateral eye patches. A surgeon who plans to use a rather prominent scleral buckle may prefer not to encourage the absorption of subretinal fluid, in which case bilateral patching would not be advised. However, if a nondrainage surgical procedure is being considered, there is some justification for the use of bilateral patching before surgery to encourage the absorption of subretinal fluid. If a superior bullous detachment is close to an attached macula, it would be wise to order bilateral patches and strict bed rest with no sitting up, while preparations are made for prompt surgery.

Most current systemic medications should be ordered preoperatively and postoperatively. Medications can be taken on the morning of surgery with a sip of water. Discontinuation of certain medications, such as anticoagulants, should be considered in consultation with the internist. Insulin doses are modified to accommodate the NPO status. Some patients appreciate a tranquilizer, especially if they are bilaterally patched.

General anesthesia is frequently used for retinal reattachment surgery, but local anesthesia is usually satisfactory, especially in primary operations. Patients to be operated with local anesthesia may be prepared with preoperative sedative, tranquilizer, or narcotic drugs.

It is helpful to have the postoperative instruction sheet placed in the bedside box on admission so that the patient's family can review it during the hospitalization and ask questions prior to discharge.

4-3

PREOPERATIVE COMPLICATIONS

Certain complications that may arise preoperatively require special attention and may delay retinal surgery.

4-3-1 Poor Visualization of Retina

Adequate visualization of the retina may be complicated by miosis or by opacities of the cornea, lens, or vitreous.

4-3-1-1 Miosis The pupil may not dilate adequately in aphakia, after prolonged use of miotic drugs, or in the presence of posterior synechiae. An 8- or 9-mm pupil is ideal, but the retina can generally be adequately examined through a 3- or 4-mm pupil. Use of a small-pupil indirect ophthalmoscope can be helpful in working through a miotic pupil.

Scleral indentation readily brings the periphery into view if the intraocular pressure is low. Generally, the pressure decreases adequately with repeated scleral indentation. But if glaucoma is present along with a small pupil, it may be advisable to lower the intraocular pressure with an agent such as oral glycerin. Thereafter, the ora serrata can be readily brought into the line of view by indenting the softened globe.

Photocoagulation of the iris, or photomydriasis, often alleviates miosis (Figure 4-1). Argon laser photocoagulation of the iris midway between the pupillary margin and the iris root causes contraction of the dilator muscle and peaks the pupil in that meridian. Treatment in at least eight meridians usually provides an adequate pupillary opening for ophthalmoscopy. Pupillary fibrosis may be amenable to Nd:YAG laser transection.

Occasionally, miosis requires a sector iridectomy, synechialysis, or both immediately before the retinal reattachment procedure. Some surgeons feel that the effect of topical dilating drops is enhanced with a subconjunctival injection of a mydriatic–cycloplegic combination. Care sould be used with subconjunctival phenylephrine injections to avoid significant elevation in blood pressure. Some miotic pupils can be temporarily dilated with flexible translimbal iris retractors.

4-3-1-2 Corneal Opacities Corneal opacities are rarely sufficient to preclude retinal surgery, but keratoplasty should be considered if necessary. The corneal and retinal surgery may be performed at the same time, facilitated by use of a temporary keratoprosthesis during the retinal procedure.

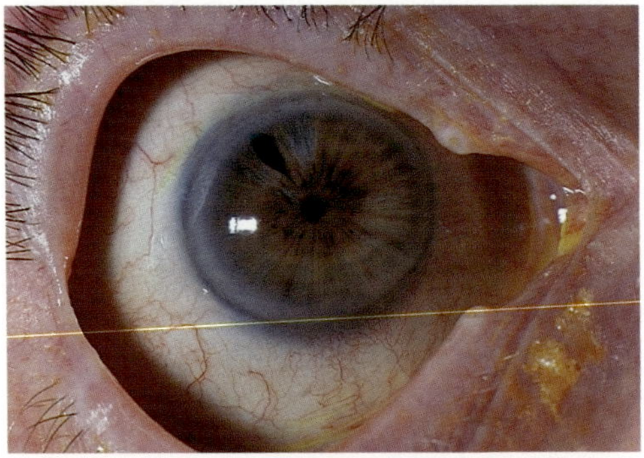

A

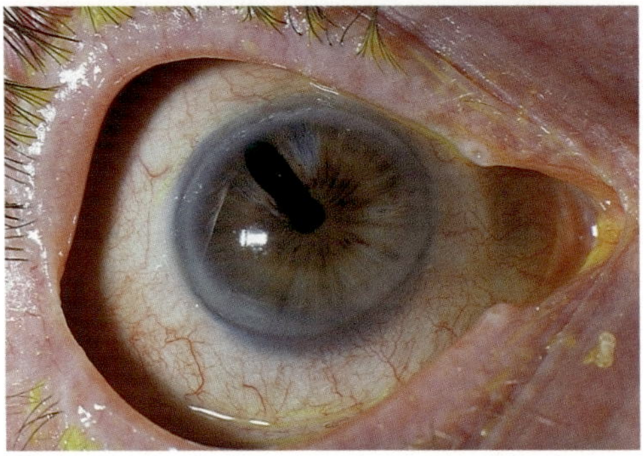

B

Figure 4-1 *Aphakic miosis. (A) Clinical photograph. (B) Same pupil immediately after enlargement with Nd:YAG laser.*
Courtesy James B. Wise, MD.

4-3-1-3 Cataract Limited opacities of the lens are common in patients with retinal detachment, but the binocular indirect ophthalmoscope usually enables adequate examination. The most common site of cortical opacities is in the inferior nasal quadrant. Fortunately, retinal breaks occur least frequently in this location. The obscuring effect of a moderate degree of nuclear sclerosis can be overcome with the indirect ophthalmoscope at maximum voltage. Extracapsular cataract surgery, which is often combined with the implantation of an intraocular lens, may compromise the visibility of the retinal periphery. If, in the presence of a significant cataract, a fairly adequate ophthalmoscopic examination is possible and reveals that the distribution of the subretinal fluid is appropriate for the apparent retinal breaks, it is generally preferable to proceed with retinal surgery without removing the cataract. Only in the occasional case of advanced cataract should the surgeon resort to cataract surgery prior to repairing the retinal detachment. In most such cases, it is appropriate to perform cataract surgery and scleral buckling at the same time.

If there is any question about the strength of the cataract wound from prior surgery, the surgeon should place additional mattress sutures across the limbus. They may be removed at the end of the scleral buckling procedure.

4-3-1-4 Vitreous Opacities Vitreous opacities, especially hemorrhage, are rather common with retinal detachment, but usually adequate examination of the retina is possible. Vitreous hemorrhage may be somewhat cleared by binocular patching and positioning the patient to allow blood to settle away from the area of the suspected retinal break. At least 48 hours should transpire before the attempt to clear the blood by patching is abandoned. If the clarity is sufficient for a retinal break that explains the detachment to be seen, it is probably best to proceed with scleral buckling instead of vitrectomy or waiting the several months required for complete clearing of vitreous hemorrhage. If the fundus cannot be seen, the eye should be examined by ultrasonography. If a retinal detachment is demonstrated, the surgeon should proceed with pars plana vitrectomy and repair of the detachment.

4-3-2 External Disease

Retinal surgery is not recommended in the presence of infection. Most retinal detachments can be deferred for several days until external infection is brought under control with appropriate antibiotic therapy. Postponement may not be necessary for mild blepharitis.

4-3-3 Glaucoma

Preoperative gonioscopy is indicated when a history, signs, or symptoms of elevated intraocular pressure exist. The presence of open-angle glaucoma prior to retinal detachment generally poses no problem. Miotics should be withheld. The ocular hypotensive effect of the detachment frequently allows discontinuance of the miotic drops for a few weeks. If, however, the pressure becomes elevated, acetazolamide (Diamox), timolol, or epinephrine may be employed. In the rare cases in which this treatment is insufficient, hyperosmotic agents may be added.

Although retinal detachment usually produces a modest degree of hypotony, in rare cases the detachment causes secondary elevation of the intraocular pressure, which tends to be refractory to any treatment until the retina is reattached (Schwartz syndrome). In the absence of significant trabecular damage from uveitis, the intraocular pressure normalizes postoperatively.

4-3-4 Uveitis

A minimal degree of flare and cells in the anterior chamber is common in retinal detachment and requires no medical treatment. Marked uveitis, however, should be vigorously treated with cycloplegic drops as well as topical and/or systemic corticosteroids as indicated. Surgery is usually delayed for a few days. Of course, care must be taken to ensure that a rhegmatogenous retinal detachment is indeed present and to rule out a nonrhegmatogenous detachment secondary to uveitis.

4-3-5 Choroidal Detachment

Retinal detachment must always be differentiated from choroidal detachment, especially in patients who have recently undergone intraocular surgery or other ocular trauma. However, rhegmatogenous retinal detachment and choroidal detachment occasionally coexist. The choroidal detachment is generally associated with hypotony, which induces further choroidal detachment, perpetuating the cycle. Such eyes often have significant uveitis as well.

The anatomic results of retinal reattachment surgery in the presence of choroidal detachment and uveitis are poor, due to a relatively high incidence of postoperative proliferative vitreoretinopathy. In such cases, treatment with systemic and topical corticosteroids for 1 or 2 weeks is sometimes beneficial, but prolonged deferment of the retinal surgery is not recommended. If the choroidal detachment is not in the area of the retinal break, the surgeon should simply proceed with retinal surgery. If, however, the choroidal detachment is in the area of the retinal break or in the area where subretinal fluid must be drained, the surgeon should begin the operation with drainage of the suprachoroidal fluid. Normal intraocular pressure can be maintained during drainage with use of a pars plana cannula for the continuous infusion of balanced salt solution into the vitreous cavity. The surgeon may then proceed immediately with conventional retinal reattachment surgery.

SUGGESTED READINGS

Michels RG, Wilkinson CP, Rice TA: *Retinal Detachment.* St Louis: CV Mosby Co; 1990.

Schepens CL: *Retinal Detachment and Allied Diseases.* Philadelphia: WB Saunders Co; 1983: vols 1, 2.

CHAPTER 5

Prophylactic Procedures

The selection of cases that may benefit from prophylactic surgery is a constantly changing frontier with widespread controversy. According to a 1994 Preferred Practice Pattern developed by the American Academy of Ophthalmology, all symptomatic retinal breaks should be treated. The selection of asymptomatic breaks to treat is summarized in Table 5-1.

5-1

INDICATIONS FOR PROPHYLACTIC TREATMENT

Retinal detachment is an uncommon disease, affecting approximately 1 in 15,000 people in the general population per year or an estimated 0.3% over a lifetime. But the incidence of retinal breaks is considerably higher, affecting 5% to 7% of the population. Some retinal breaks have minimal, if any, risk for the possible development of a retinal detachment. This includes macular holes that occur as a degenerative process in elderly patients and asymptomatic, small, round atrophic holes near the ora serrata, particularly in phakic patients. However, equatorial horseshoe tears with relevant symptoms progress to retinal detachment in about one third of cases. Most surgeons agree that a large horseshoe tear near the equator in the superior temporal quadrant, with symptoms of flashes and floaters and with associated vitreous hemorrhage, should be treated prophylactically to avoid retinal detachment. In contrast, most would not advise treatment of a small, round atrophic hole near the inferior ora serrata in an asymptomatic patient. Between these two obvious examples lies a broad spectrum of retinal breaks for which the surgeon must exercise judgment about instituting prophylactic treatment.

Most of the breaks reported in surveys of asymptomatic patients or in autopsy series are of the atrophic type, and only a small proportion are horseshoe tears. There is no general rule for the selection of patients for treatment. Each case

TABLE 5-1

Indications for Treatment of Retinal Tears and Holes in Asymptomatic Patients

Type of Tear or Hole	Phakia	High Myopia	Status of Other Eye*	Aphakia or Pseudophakia	Prior to Cataract Surgery
Atrophic hole	Rarely	Rarely	Rarely	Rarely	Rarely
Operculated hole	No	Rarely	Rarely	Rarely	Rarely
Lattice degeneration with or without hole	No	Rarely	Sometimes	Rarely	Rarely
Horseshoe tear	Sometimes	Sometimes	Frequently	Frequently	Frequently
Subclinical retinal detachment	Sometimes	Frequently	Frequently	Frequently	Frequently
Dialysis	Almost always	Almost always	Almost always	Almost always	Almost always

**Applies to patients who have had a retinal detachment in the other eye.*

Source: Adapted from Precursors of Rhegmatogenous Retinal Detachment in Adults. *Preferred Practice Pattern. San Francisco: American Academy of Ophthalmology; 1994.*

should be judged on its own characteristics. The surgeon can make a decision only after a balanced consideration of multiple variables, including

1. Symptoms
2. Location, type, size, and apparent age of break
3. Presence or absence of subretinal fluid
4. Vitreous hemorrhage
5. Aphakia or pseudophakia
6. Refractive error
7. Status of other eye
8. Patient's age
9. Family history
10. Patient's life expectancy and occupation
11. Any anticipated cataract surgery

Each of these factors should be carefully evaluated before a final decision is made.

5-1-1 Symptoms

The presence of relevant symptoms, such as flashes and floaters, suggests the need for prophylactic surgery. However, care must be taken to rule out irrelevant symptoms. Certainly, common vitreous floaters in the presence of a small atrophic hole would not be regarded as relevant, nor would the flashes of migraine.

5-1-2 Location and Size of Break

Generally, the risk of subsequent retinal detachment is higher for retinal breaks that are above the horizontal meridian. The tendency is to advise treatment for superior temporal breaks, because detachment is likely to cause macular detachment more quickly. Concern is increased if the break is at the equator or posterior to the equator. This concern is based on the fact that very anterior breaks near the ora are often covered and protected by the vitreous base, whereas an unprotected posterior break causing retinal detachment is apt to progress into the macula rapidly. Furthermore, detachments caused by posterior breaks are more difficult to cure. A surgeon would be more inclined to operate prophylactically on a large retinal tear than on a small break and would certainly treat all giant tears. If vitreous traction on the break is marked, as manifested by a highly elevated flap or by the posterior margin of the tear being somewhat rolled posteriorly, some form of prophylaxis is well advised.

5-1-3 Age of Break

The exact age of a tear cannot always be determined. When associated vitreous hemorrhage is present or there are symptoms of flashes and floaters, it may be assumed that the break occurred recently. But if there is secondary surrounding hyperplasia of the retinal pigment epithelium, the break is old. If the break has been present for more than 1 month without causing retinal detachment, the risk of detachment seems to be much less than for recent breaks. Regarding pigment, it is necessary to differentiate reactive pigmentation surrounding a break from pigment that is seen beneath the break at the level of the choroid and on the flap of the tear. The latter predates the development of the break and probably represents a preexisting site of vitreoretinal adhesion. The type of pigmentation that develops around a retinal tear, which may be regarded as a small demarcation line, has great significance by suggesting that the break has been present for several months or longer.

5-1-4 Presence of Fluid

Although the presence of subretinal fluid technically justifies use of the term *retinal detachment*, a small amount of fluid in an otherwise low-risk break, such as the round atrophic hole of lattice degeneration, is not necessarily a compelling reason for treatment. Many surgeons believe that the presence of fluid is an indication for surgery if the fluid has extended more than 1 disc diameter away from the edge of the break. But if the fluid appears static in extent, as evidenced by a demarcation line, observation without intervention is appropriate.

5-1-5 Vitreous Hemorrhage

Most retinal tears that produce vitreous hemorrhage should be treated, especially if there is traction on a retinal vessel.

5-1-6 Aphakia or Pseudophakia

Because the prevalence of retinal detachment is much higher in the aphakic/pseudophakic population, breaks in such eyes are assumed to have a relatively greater risk of detachment. If an immature cataract is present but the retinal periphery can still be visualized with binocular indirect ophthalmoscopy and scleral indentation, it may be prudent to treat high-risk retinal breaks disclosed by this technique prior to cataract extraction.

5-1-7 Myopia

The risk of retinal detachment is considerably greater in cases of high myopia. Therefore, the benefit of prophylactic surgery to reduce the risk of detachment may be greater for a myopic eye than for an emmetropic eye with a similar break.

5-1-8 Status of Other Eye

The status of the other eye is important. If a retinal detachment had occurred in the other eye, the surgeon is more likely to decide that breaks in this eye should be treated prophylactically.

5-1-9 History

If the family has a significant history of retinal detachment, the tendency to recommend treatment is usually greater. If the patient has a short life expectancy, treatment should be discouraged. If there is some likelihood of future trauma due to the patient's occupation, travel to remote destinations, or unreliable followup, a surgeon is more disposed to intervene.

5-1-10 Lesions Without Breaks

Occasionally, decisions similar to those in regard to retinal breaks without detachment are necessary for lesions without breaks that have the potential for developing breaks. The question most commonly arises for lattice degeneration. Prophylactic treatment of lattice degeneration without breaks usually is not recommended, even if cataract surgery is anticipated.

Most patients with retinoschisis should not be treated but should be observed periodically. Unusual indications for treating the retinoschisis patient include associated retinal detachment, vitreous hemorrhage, and the very rare threat of extension of schisis into the macula. The question of treating outer-layer breaks with little or no subretinal fluid is controversial. Some surgeons favor treatment but most prefer to withhold therapy unless the beginning of retinal detachment is documented.

Although a small break in peripheral cystoid degeneration does in rare instances lead to retinal detachment, the occurrence is far too uncommon to justify prophylactic treatment for the ubiquitous entity of peripheral cystoid degeneration.

5-2

PROPHYLACTIC TECHNIQUES

Diathermy, cryotherapy, photocoagulation, and, in certain rare instances, scleral buckling have all been used for prophylactic treatment of retinal breaks without detachment. Diathermy is infrequently used at present because of the need for conjunctival peritomy, but good results can certainly be obtained with it. Whereas scleral-buckling procedures are generally performed in the operating room, most cryotherapy or photocoagulation procedures are performed in the outpatient department or office.

The choice of treatment technique depends on the surgeon's experience and the availability of equipment; however, the anteroposterior location of the retinal tear is the primary determinant. In general, far anterior tears are treated with cryotherapy, posterior tears with photocoagulation, and intermediate tears with either modality. Recently, however, the laser indirect ophthalmoscope (LIO) with scleral indentation is a frequent choice for very anterior breaks.

5-2-1 Cryotherapy

Good anesthesia is obtained by supplementing topical 4% lidocaine with an injection of subconjunctival 1% lidocaine in the involved quadrants. Retrobulbar anesthesia is not recommended, because the patient then loses the ability to position the eye in accordance with the surgeon's instructions.

To apply cryotherapy for a retinal break near the ora, the surgeon instructs the patient to move the eye in the direction of the break. Breaks near the equator are most easily indented with the cryoprobe when the eye is approximately in the primary position. Breaks posterior to the equator can often be reached with the cryoprobe if the patient is instructed to move the eye away from the meridian of the break and toward the surgeon, who is positioned in the meridian opposite that of the break.

A number of applications should be used to surround the break completely with an adequate margin. For large breaks, an attempt should be made to avoid freezing the exposed pigment epithelium within the tear, because this will encourage the migration of retinal pigment epithelial cells into the vitreous. In a patient with lattice degeneration, the treatment should include not only the lattice patch but also adjacent normal retina on all sides of the patch. More posterior lesions can be reached by a small incision in the conjunctiva.

The eye should be patched for a few hours until the effects of anesthesia have dissipated. In the case of horseshoe tears, the patient is generally restricted in activities until some pigmentation appears around the break, which generally occurs within 7 to 10 days.

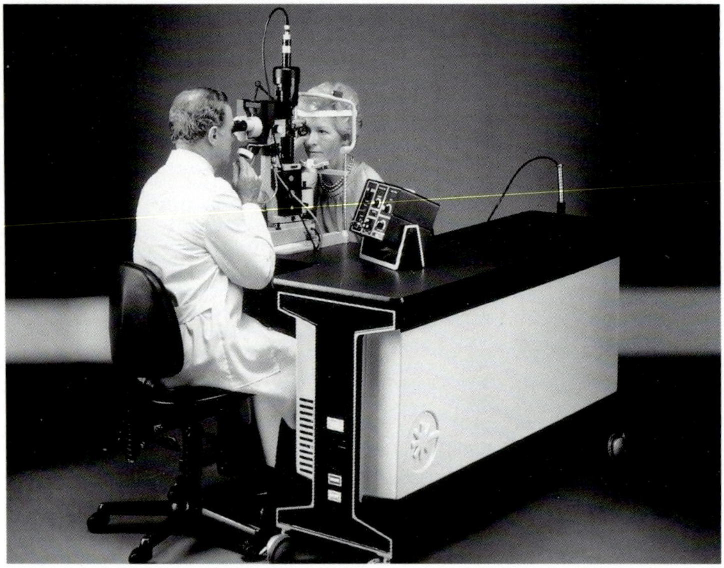

Figure 5-1 *Coherent laser photocoagulator, one of several currently available laser photocoagulators.* *Courtesy Coherent, Inc.*

5-2-2 Photocoagulation

For various reasons, including the possible liberation of viable retinal pigment epithelial cells during cryopexy, there is a theoretical advantage to photocoagulation over cryopexy, using the xenon arc, argon laser, or diode laser (Figure 5-1). A laser photocoagulator provides an excellent viewing system, with either the laser indirect ophthalmoscope (LIO) or the binocular biomicroscope and slit lamp used in association with the Goldmann three-mirror or panfunduscopic contact lens. The entire retinal break should be surrounded by a series of photocoagulation lesions. The appropriate end point for these lesions is the development of a white reaction within the retina.

The troublesome problem of recurrent vitreous hemorrhages due to avulsion of a retinal vessel at the site of the break may be an indication for a buckling procedure or vitrectomy, if photocoagulation of the vessel has been unsuccessful in stopping the bleeding.

5-3

RESULTS OF PROPHYLACTIC TREATMENT

The efficacy of prophylactic treatment obviously depends on the relative risk of detachment specific to the entity. The usual purpose of prophylactic treatment is to prevent development of a retinal detachment, and this has been accomplished in more than 90% of the treated patients in most series. If a retinal detachment ensues within 1 day after a prophylactic procedure, it might be argued that the treatment actually precipitated the detachment. But the detachment could very well be due to progression of the disease despite treatment. If such an event occurs, the detachment can usually be successfully treated by a scleral-buckling procedure. If the detachment develops several weeks later, it is more likely due to the ongoing, progressive nature of the basic disease and is not to be regarded as an iatrogenic complication. While some detachments are caused by the treated breaks, in other cases detachment subsequent to treatment is due to a new break in a different meridian.

5-4

COMPLICATIONS OF PROPHYLACTIC TREATMENT

The most significant complication of prophylactic treatment is macular fibrosis, which develops in most instances within weeks after treatment. This entity, also referred to as *macular pucker*, may be due to the progression of the basic disease process or it may be a complication of the treatment. Fortunately, such complications are infrequent. It may be safely concluded that prophylactic treatment is free of complications in the vast majority of cases.

Pathogenetic mechanisms leading to, or associated with, the retinal tear itself (such as posterior vitreous detachment or vitreous hemorrhage) can also initiate macular epiretinal fibrosis. Vitreous hemorrhage after prophylactic treatment is rare, except where there is associated avulsion of a retinal vessel. Occasionally, new retinal breaks develop within a few days or weeks after prophylaxis. Some of these occur at the site of treatment, but often they occur in untreated areas and almost exclusively in eyes that initially had horseshoe tears.

SUGGESTED READINGS

Banks WS III, Havener WH: Unanticipated posterior freezing: a hazard in retinal cryosurgery. *Trans Am Acad Ophthalmol Otolaryngol* 1970;74:80–84.

Byer NE: Cystic retinal tufts and their relationship to retinal detachment. *Arch Ophthalmol* 1981;99:1788–1790.

Byer NE: Lattice degeneration of the retina. *Surv Ophthalmol* 1979;23:213–248.

Byer NE: Long-term natural history study of senile retinoschisis with implications for management. *Ophthalmology* 1986;93:1127–1137.

Byer NE: The natural history of asymptomatic retinal breaks. *Ophthalmology* 1982;89: 1033–1039.

Byer NE: *The Peripheral Retina in Profile: A Stereoscopic Atlas.* Torrance, CA: Criterion Press; 1982.

Combs JL, Welch RB: Retinal breaks without detachment: natural history, management and long-term follow-up. *Trans Am Ophthalmol Soc* 1982;80:64–97.

Davis MD: Natural history of retinal breaks without detachment. *Arch Ophthalmol* 1974; 92:183–184.

Dobbie JG: Cryotherapy in the management of senile retinoschisis. *Trans Am Acad Ophthalmol Otolaryngol* 1969;73:1047–1060.

Dumas J, Schepens CL: Chorioretinal lesions predisposing to retinal breaks. *Am J Ophthalmol* 1966;61:620–630.

Foos RY: Tears of the peripheral retina: pathogenesis, incidence and classification in autopsy eyes. *Mod Probl Ophthalmol* 1975;15:68–81.

Hagler WS, Woldoff HS: Retinal detachment in relation to senile retinoschisis. *Trans Am Acad Ophthalmol Otolaryngol* 1973;77:OP99–113.

Hirose T, Marcil G, Schepens CL, et al: Acquired retinoschisis: observations and treatment. In: Pruett RC, Regan CDJ, eds: *Retinal Congress*. New York: Appleton-Century-Crofts; 1972:489–504.

Kramer SG, Benson WE: Prophylactic therapy of retinal breaks. *Surv Ophthalmol* 1977;22: 41–47.

Precursors of Rhegmatogenous Retinal Detachment in Adults. Preferred Practice Pattern. San Francisco: American Academy of Ophthalmology; 1994.

Roseman RC, Olk RJ, Arribas NP, et al: Limited retinal detachment: a retrospective analysis of treatment with transconjunctival retinocryopexy. *Ophthalmology* 1986;93:216–233.

Schepens CL: *Retinal Detachment and Allied Diseases*. Philadelphia: WB Saunders Co; 1983: vols 1, 2.

Sigelman J: Vitreous base classification of retinal tears: clinical application. *Surv Ophthalmol* 1980;25:59–70.

Smiddy WE, Flynn HW, Nicholson DH, et al: Results and complications in treated retinal breaks. *Am J Ophthalmol* 1991;98:1769–1775.

Straatsma BR, Foos RY: Typical and reticular degenerative retinoschisis. XXVI Francis I. Proctor Memorial Lecture. *Am J Ophthalmol* 1973;75:551–575.

Straatsma BR, Zeegen PD, Foos RY, et al: Lattice degeneration of the retina. XXX Edward Jackson Memorial Lecture. *Trans Am Acad Ophthalmol Otolaryngol* 1974;78:OP87–113.

CHAPTER 6

Retinal Reattachment Surgery

Inflammatory detachments are usually treated medically. Some serous detachments, such as choroidal hemangioma, respond to photocoagulation. Selected traction detachments, such as diabetic or posttraumatic detachments, may be cured with intraocular microsurgery. Radiation therapy is often used for detachments secondary to metastatic tumors. This chapter is confined to the surgical management of rhegmatogenous detachments.

Controversy exists regarding the details of the surgical technique, but surgeons generally agree on the three basic steps in closing retinal breaks and reattaching the retina.

1. Conducting a thorough preoperative examination with the goal of identifying all retinal breaks and assessing any vitreous traction on the retina

2. Creating a controlled injury to the retinal pigment epithelium and retina to produce a chorioretinal adhesion at the site of all retinal breaks

3. Employing an appropriate technique, such as scleral buckling and/or intravitreal gas, to approximate the retinal breaks to the underlying treated retinal pigment epithelium

If the surgeon follows these basics and applies modern surgical techniques, retinal reattachment may be expected in more than 85% of all cases and in 95% of uncomplicated primary detachments.

The traditional scleral buckle has served very well for more than 40 years. Recent developments have produced a comprehensive menu for retinal reattachment surgery from which the surgeon may select the appropriate procedure for each case (Table 6-1). A permanent scleral buckle is still indicated in more than half of all detachments, but the other alternatives are appropriately indicated for the resolution of specific problems.

TABLE 6-1

A Menu for Retinal Reattachment Surgery

Procedure	Sample Indications
Photocoagulation of retina	Small detachment—2 to 4 disc diameters (see Section 6-2-1)
Transconjunctival cryotherapy of retina	Small detachment if media are not clear enough for photocoagulation, but clear enough to see break (see Section 6-2-2)
Pneumatic retinopexy	Detachment with superior break without proliferative vitreoretinopathy (see Section 6-2-3)
Temporary scleral buckle (gelatin or balloon)	Detachment with inferior dialysis in child (gelatin) or inferior break in adult (balloon) (see Sections 6-2-4 and 6-2-5)
Permanent scleral buckle	Detachment with multiple breaks with or without moderate proliferative vitreoretinopathy (see Section 6-1)
Vitrectomy	Prominent proliferative vitreoretinopathy or diabetic traction detachment (see Section 6-3)

Temporary scleral buckling with scleral infolding, gelatin, or orbital ballon is always designated with the appropriate adjective. But the term *scleral buckling* without a qualifying adjective is generally recognized as referring to a permanent scleral buckle with the implantation of a foreign material.

6-1

SCLERAL BUCKLING PROCEDURE

For scleral buckling, the face, eyelids, and conjunctiva are prepared with appropriate antiseptic techniques, and the drapes are applied. Various techniques of draping are available, but it should be recognized that the eyelid margins are the part of the operative field most susceptible to infection. Therefore, a plastic adhesive drape placed over the opened lids so that the drape adheres to the eyelids and adjacent part of the face is recommended. An incision is made in the plastic drape in the plane of the palpebral fissure, and the free margins of the cut drape are rolled posteriorly over the lid margins and held securely in place with the eyelid speculum. Many types of speculums have been successfully used, but the simple wire speculum of Barraquer has been found to be very satisfactory. A colored drape should be placed over the head and body to supplement the plastic drape. The colored drape minimizes the glare of reflected light and absorbs excess irrigating fluid.

6-1-1 Opening Incision

The classic opening incision for retinal detachment surgery has traditionally been circumferential and 5 or 6 mm posterior to the limbus, but in recent years a limbal conjunctival peritomy has gained interest.

The conjunctiva and Tenon's capsule are fused together at the limbus, so that both tissues can be incised together. The limbal incision is easy and quick, provides good coverage of any implanted buckling material, and facilitates rapid closure. The peritomy is supplemented by two relaxing incisions perpendicular to the limbus (Figure 6-1). Although a complete peritomy is frequently employed, a partial peritomy may be sufficient for a limited detachment. Adequate exposure for a quadrantic detachment can be achieved by a peritomy covering five hours of the clock, which would expose the two rectus muscles bordering the involved quadrant.

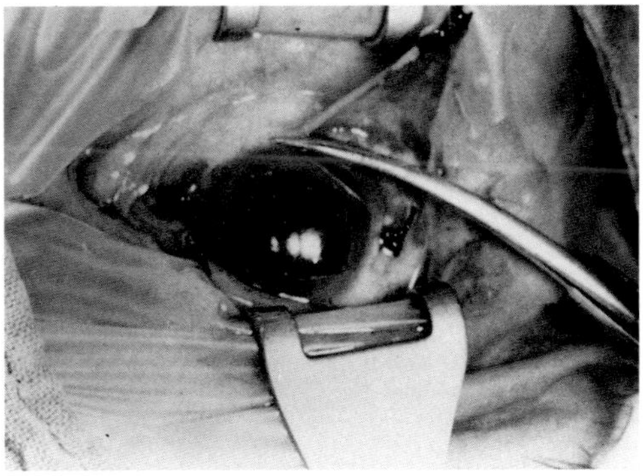

Figure 6-1 *Limbal peritomy. (Black sutures used to mark four corners of two horizontal relaxing incisions are for illustration only and are not required during surgery.)*

Traction sutures should be placed beneath the insertions of the rectus muscles to facilitate positioning the globe. Rather heavy suture material, such as No. 2-0, is recommended to give the assistant surgeon substantial bulk for gripping. The suture may be passed through the hole of a fenestrated muscle hook, which is then passed under the rectus muscle (Figure 6-2). The suture is drawn through the fenestration with toothed forceps as the muscle hook is withdrawn. The two free ends of this suture are tied together at approximately 4 cm and 15 cm from the globe. Four traction sutures provide adequate means for orientation of the globe. Alternatively, the suture can be passed beneath the muscle with the use of a curved or angled hemostat. Or the surgeon can grasp the tip of a swagged-on needle and lead the suture beneath the muscle by passing the blunt end of the needle backward beneath the muscle, where it can be picked up with forceps. If a partial peritomy is used, only the exposed muscles need be secured in this fashion, while the other

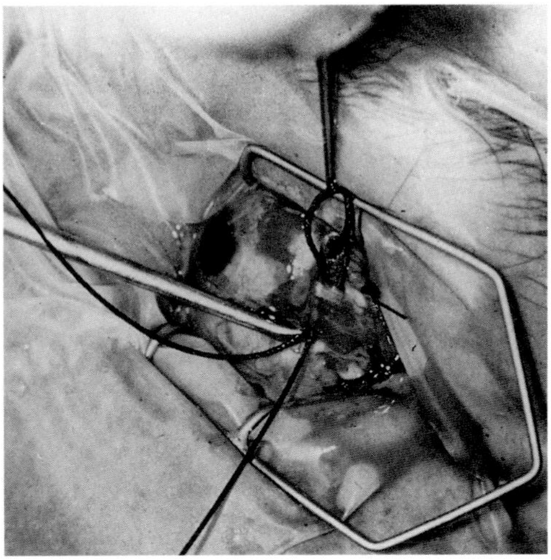

Figure 6-2 *Fenestrated muscle hook used to pass traction suture beneath rectus muscle.*

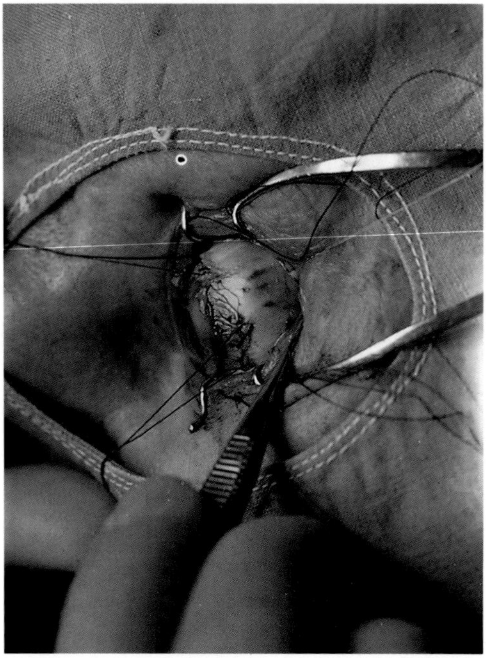

Figure 6-3 *Three radial scleral dehiscences of superior temporal equatorial zone.*

Reproduced with permission from Watzke RC: Scleral staphylomas and retinal detachment. Arch Ophthalmol *1963;70:796–804. Copyright 1963 American Medical Association.*

rectus muscles can be secured by passing a needle through the conjunctiva and muscle insertion.

After all four rectus muscles are secured with traction sutures, the sclera should be examined. It can be exposed for inspection by rotating the globe with two adjacent traction sutures and pushing the intermuscular fascia posteriorly with a cotton-tipped applicator. The examination is repeated for all open quadrants. The surgeon should look for abnormalities such as anomalous vortex veins or scleral thinning. Thinning may be manifested by a gray color within a certain geographic zone, which is the underlying choroid; more often, thinning is manifested by radial gray lines in the equatorial or preequatorial area. These lines are most common in the superior temporal quadrant and are called *radial staphylomas*, *scleral cracks*, or *scleral dehiscences* (Figure 6-3).

After examination of the sclera, the surgeon should examine the retina, 360°, with binocular indirect ophthalmoscopy and scleral indentation. The investment of a few minutes at this time will pay dividends. Important lesions that were not disclosed preoperatively may become apparent, and occasionally this examination reveals significant changes that have developed since the preoperative examination.

6-1-2 Localization of Breaks

A localizing mark is made on the sclera, overlaying the posterior edge of all retinal breaks. If a break is large, additional marks should be placed at the anterior and lateral margins. Localizing marks are important guides for placement of the buckle. If all the diathermy or cryotherapy is not applied with ophthalmoscopic monitoring, the marks also serve as orientation points for additional treatment.

The technique of direct localization involves observing the break with the binocular indirect ophthalmoscope. As the surgeon notes each retinal break, a marking instrument is pressed against the globe and the resultant scleral indentation is oriented to coincide with the posterior edge of the break. Scleral indentation can be accomplished with a flat diathermy electrode. When the electrode is in position, a burn is applied that marks both the sclera and the retina. The marking is easily performed if the detachment is sufficiently flat to allow the retinal pigment epithelium to be pressed inward against the sensory retina. If the detachment is high and bullous, this is not possible and the surgeon must try to compensate for the parallax effect. With bullous detachments, the tendency is to localize the break too far posteriorly. If the surgeon is aware of the problem, an adequate anterior compensation can be made.

Various other localization techniques in addition to diathermy are available. The cryosurgical probe can be used, and the temporary freezing mark it produces on the sclera can be marked with a sterile felt-tipped pen or with a cautery. Various indentation marking devices are also available, including the thimble device of Gass and the scleral localizers of Urrets-Zavalia or O'Connor. The tip of the scleral marker is firmly pressed against the eye for a few seconds, and the pressure creates a temporary black mark on the sclera (Figure 6-4). In still another method, the

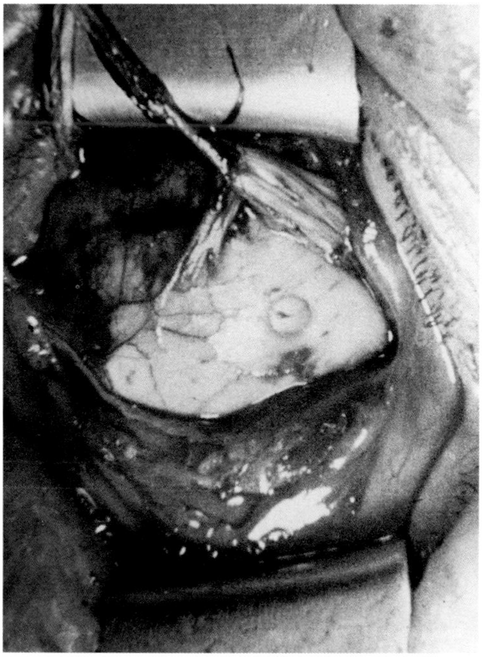

Figure 6-4 *Annular localizing mark produced with pressure-type scleral marker.*

surgeon estimates the approximate location of the break and grasps the sclera with toothed forceps, which are used for scleral indentation. The forceps can be repositioned as many times as necessary to bring them to the proper location. The temporary marks produced can be transformed into permanent ones with ink or with superficial cautery of the sclera. All of these methods have been successfully used, but each should be used with caution over thin sclera. Occasionally, the localization coincides with some definite landmark on the surface of the sclera, such as an episcleral vessel, a vortex vein, or a muscle insertion. With such a clearcut landmark, an additional mark is not necessary.

6-1-3 Thermal Treatment

A variety of methods have been employed to irritate the choroid and pigment epithelium so that they form chorioretinal adhesions to seal retinal breaks. A partial list of methods includes puncture with cautery, superficial cauterization, electrolysis, and irritative chemicals, such as sodium hydroxide, caustic potash, carbolic acid, and tincture of iodine. The three most popular techniques, which have persisted for many years, are diathermy, cryotherapy, and photocoagulation.

6-1-3-1 Diathermy Diathermy should be applied through thinned sclera, beneath partial-thickness scleral flaps. This technique avoids full-thickness destruction of sclera and achieves a more uniform diathermy reaction at the level of the choroid and retinal pigment epithelium. The surgeon may apply the diathermy while inspecting the retina with the ophthalmoscope and limit the intensity of diathermy to that required to produce a moderately white lesion in the retina. On the other hand, the surgeon may elect to apply the diathermy without ophthalmoscopic control. An experienced surgeon can predict the probable ophthalmoscopic result on the basis of the scleral reaction. The diathermy burns are not contiguous but are spaced approximately 1.5 mm apart. The resultant lesions produce intermittent pigmentary changes in the fundus that have been referred to as "leopard skin."

Numerous diathermy instruments are available, such as the Walker unit, the Bovie unit, and the Medical Instruments Research Associates (MIRA) unit (Figure 6-5). Various types of diathermy tips can be used: a 2-mm pin for perforation and release of subretinal fluid, a conical tip or a small flat tip for surface diathermy, and a large flat tip for localization. Diathermy leaves a permanent mark both on the surface of the sclera and in the fundus, thereby enabling identification of all treated areas. Because of the destructive nature of diathermy lesions, care must be taken not to treat in the horizontal meridians, where the long posterior ciliary artery, nerve, or both might be inadvertently destroyed.

6-1-3-2 Cryotherapy The use of cryotherapy has gained in popularity since its reintroduction in 1964. A survey of retinal surgeons revealed that the majority of surgeons now employ it for most cases. Although it is possible to apply cryotherapy beneath partial-thickness scleral flaps, it is not necessary to do so. Cryotherapy can be used through full-thickness sclera without significant scleral damage.

The goal of cryotherapy is to apply contiguous lesions completely surrounding each retinal break. Cryotherapy can be applied while observing the fundus with the ophthalmoscope, and the freezing is generally terminated when the surgeon observes the appearance of an ice ball in the plane of the neurosensory retina. A prominent white change develops at the area of retinal freezing. In bullous detachments, the ice ball does not reach the retina itself, but the freezing of the retinal pigment epithelium can be discerned by a change of color to dull orange. The freezing action should be terminated approximately 1 second after the appearance of the ice ball in the fundus.

Cryotherapy application is usually monitored with the ophthalmoscope, but can also be done without monitoring. In the latter case, the surgeon applies cryotherapy to the dried surface of the sclera until an annulus of frozen sclera approximately 1 mm in width appears around the tip of the cryoprobe. The surgeon may also elect to apply cryotherapy for a specific duration, in which case several treatments should be applied with ophthalmoscopic observation as the number of seconds required to obtain the desired result is

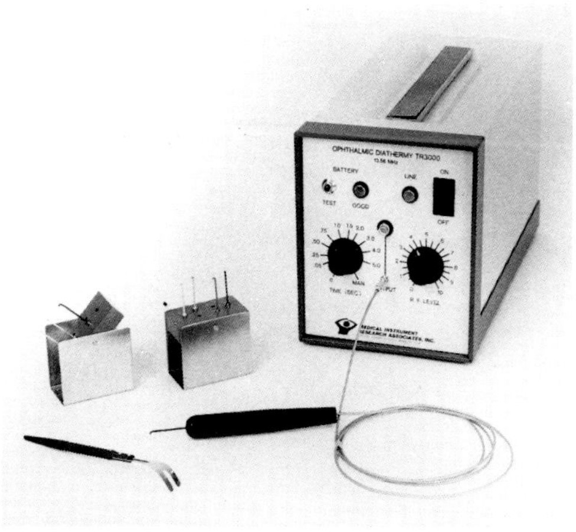

Figure 6-5 *MIRA diathermy unit, one of several currently available.*

Courtesy MIRA, Inc.

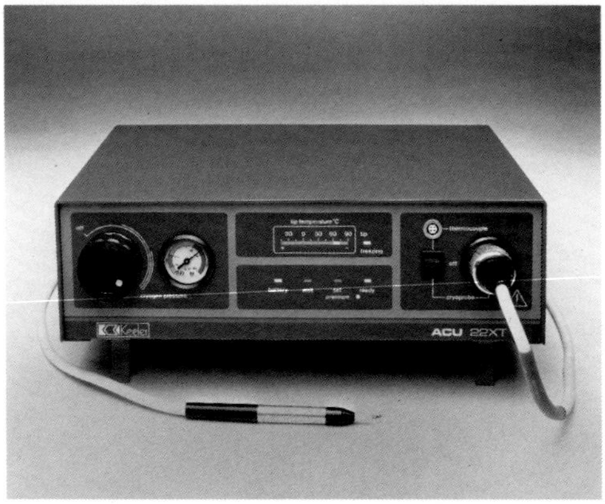

Figure 6-6 *Keeler cryosurgical unit, one of several currently available.*
Courtesy Keeler, Ltd.

noted. After the appropriate duration has been determined for a given eye, the surgeon may proceed to apply cryotherapy with that duration in other locations. However, because a longer duration is required in focal areas where the sclera or choroid is thicker, scarred, or edematous, inadequate treatment could result from using a predetermined duration without ophthalmoscopic monitoring. The surgeon must keep in mind all areas that have been treated, because no permanent mark is left on the surface of the sclera to identify a treated area and the change within the retina can be very subtle. However, in many cases, a persistent, subtle whitening of the retina allows for detecting the treated areas. The whitening is most evident about 10 minutes after freezing.

Contemporary cryosurgical units use either carbon dioxide or nitrous oxide (Figure 6-6). These units are based on the physical principle that a sudden release of high-pressure gas produces an associated drop in temperature.

The main advantages of cryosurgery are that it does not destroy sclera and it eliminates the need for dissecting scleral flaps. As a result, operating time is decreased. Moreover, sparing the sclera makes reoperation easier and safer. Cryotherapy can be used through 360°, and no significant damage to the long posterior ciliary arteries and nerves occurs. The one use of cryotherapy that has been generally accepted without controversy is for the transconjunctival treatment of peripheral retinal breaks without detachment, particularly when there is some haze of the media that would rule out the use of photocoagulation.

6-1-3-3 Photocoagulation Photocoagulation to induce adhesive lesions for retinal detachment is not widely practiced. However, the surgeon can close retinal breaks with scleral buckling or intravitreal gas and then apply photocoagulation.

6-1-4 Scleral Buckling Techniques

More than half of all retinal detachments were formerly cured without scleral buckling by the use of retinopexy, a simple diathermy and drainage procedure. However, this operation entailed prolonged hospitalization with bed rest, bilateral patching, and extensive use of pinhole spectacles. Scleral buckling was devised to relieve tractional forces and to promote early closure of retinal breaks. Its introduction represented an advance, allowing early ambulation, decreased hospitalization, and a marked increase in the anatomic cure rate. But scleral buckling has given rise to a new set of complications, including infection, erosion of the implant material into the globe, and extrusion of the material through the conjunctiva. As a result of recent advances, these complications have been minimized and scleral buckling is now widely accepted. Several procedures are available:

1. Scleral surgery without implant (now used very rarely)
   - Full-thickness scleral resection (no longer used for rhegmatogenous retinal detachment)
   - Lamellar scleral resection (very rarely used)
   - Circumferential scleral infolding
   - Radial scleral infolding
   - Scleral outfolding
2. Scleral buckling with implant, either segmental or encircling
   - Intrascleral
   - Episcleral

6-1-4-1 Scleral Infolding The circumferential scleral infolding developed by Chamlin was popularized by Pischel (Figure 6-7A). In this procedure, two incisions are made parallel to the limbus, about 3 to 4 mm apart. The incision depth is approximately two thirds of the thickness of the sclera. Mattress sutures are placed through the lips of the wound, then subretinal fluid is drained. As the mattress sutures are securely tied, the sclera between the parallel incisions is folded into the eye, creating a moderately prominent buckle with circumferential orientation. Although the procedure is not widely employed at present, it is still useful for creating a temporary scleral buckle near the ora without the use of foreign material. The buckling effect usually lasts 2 or 3 months, which is adequate for most breaks.

The scleral infolding procedure of Sanchez-Bulnes, and its modifications, involve two or more radial scleral incisions. Approximation of the incisions creates a localized scleral pucker to produce a circumferential fold between the two pairs of sutured incisions (Figure 6-7B). With several such incisions, the buckling effect can

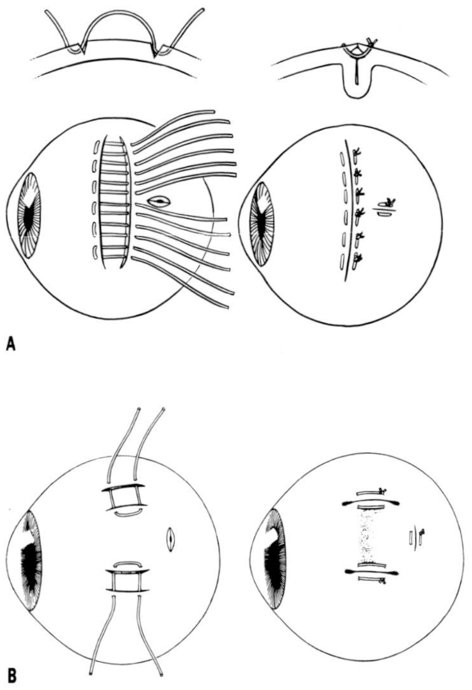

Figure 6-7 *Scleral infolding operation. (A) Circumferential. (B) Radial.*

be extended over several hours of the clock. The procedure is not widely used in the United States at this time, but some surgeons find it to be a useful adjunct to the standard buckling procedures, particularly for the creation of a relatively low temporary buckle near the ora.

6-1-4-2 Implant Materials Various materials have been used for scleral buckling, including fascia lata, palmaris tendon, plantaris tendon, knee cartilage, donor sclera, dura mater, polyviol, polyethylene, encircling nonabsorbable sutures, encircling absorbable sutures, gelatin, hydrogel, and silicone. By far the most popular, silicone is a soft, synthetic rubber material that is nontoxic and nonallergenic. Readily available, it is produced in a variety of molded shapes that can be modified by the surgeon and used in either solid or sponge form (Figure 6-8). Implants can be placed within the sclera or on its surface. These silicone implants are safe and very different from the silicone materials used for breast implants.

6-1-4-3 Intrascleral Buckle An intrascleral buckle may be performed in a segmental fashion in order to involve only a limited part of the circumference of the globe. A scleral bed is created by lamellar dissection, an appropriate implant (such as silicone or gelatin) is placed in the bed of the undermining, and the flaps are then closed over the top with sutures. This "trap-door procedure" creates a satisfactory buckle (Figure 6-9A).

The most popular intrascleral implants make use of an encircling band (Figure 6-9B). A grooved implant of solid silicone

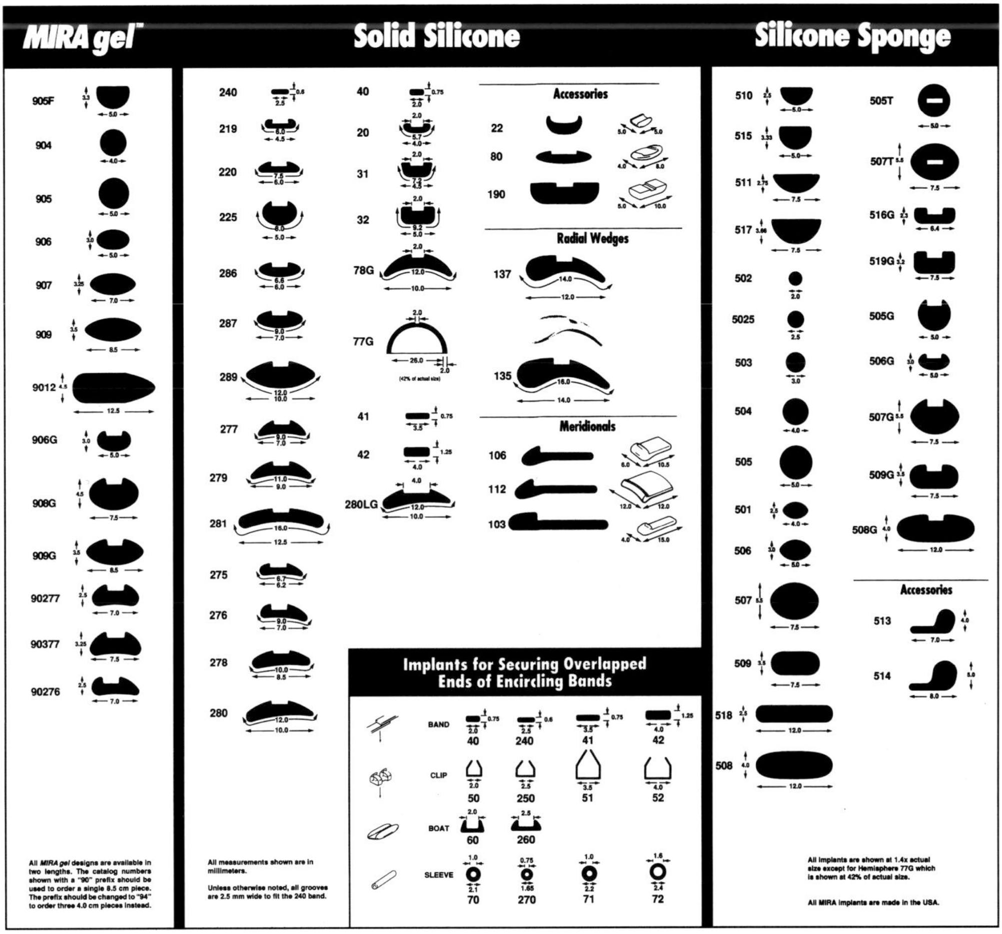

Figure 6-8 *Implants and exoplants for scleral buckling. All measurements are in millimeters. Courtesy MIRA, Inc.*

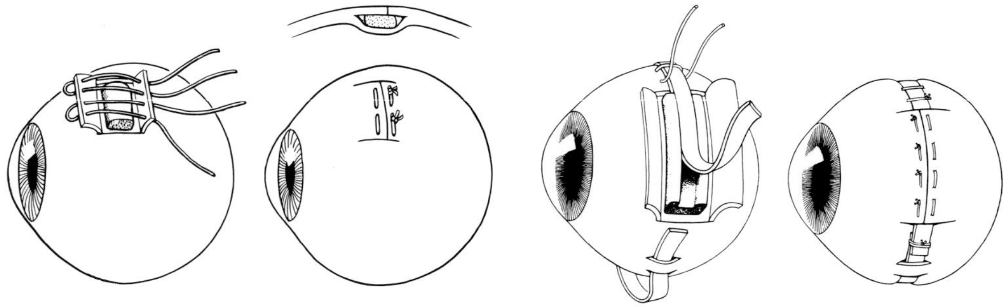

A

B

Figure 6-9 *Intrascleral buckles. (A) Trap-door procedures. (B) Implant with encircling band, which may be secured with scleral tunnel ("belt loop") or mattress suture. Band is tied to itself with clove hitch or square knot.*

is placed beneath the encircling band. The implant can be fashioned and positioned to underlie the retinal breaks and can vary in length from one to twelve hours of the clock and in width from 4 to 12 mm. The grooved implant is placed beneath scleral flaps, and the encircling band is placed on the surface of the sclera in the areas not undermined. The ends of the encircling band are joined together, with only moderate tension, by a metal clip, a suture, or a silicone sleeve. The encircling band is secured with at least one mattress suture in each quadrant where it passes over the scleral surface. Alternatively, the band may be passed through a small scleral tunnel in each quadrant (the "belt-loops procedure").

6-1-4-4 Episcleral Buckle In recent years, the use of episcleral buckling techniques has increased. A segmental buckle can be created by suturing a piece of solid silicone to the surface of the sclera, but the most popular material is silicone sponge (Figure 6-10). The sponge is commercially available in various sizes, but any of these may be modified by additional cutting. The sponge can be oriented in either a circumferential or a radial position as the nature of the retinal break dictates. Such sponges have generally been used to create segmental buckles, but an encircling buckle can also be produced with the same material.

The segmental episcleral buckling procedure is frequently accomplished without the drainage of subretinal fluid. The sponge is sutured to the surface of the globe while the assistant applies a moderate degree of stretch so that the sponge is tied down under some tension. If fluid is not drained, the intraocular pressure rises, but this elevation is temporary and is not associated with any significant ocular morbidity. The pressure may be elevated as high as 50 mm Hg, but in a nonglaucomatous eye will quickly fall to normal levels. The procedure should not be used if aqueous outflow is poor, as in open-angle glaucoma. In such cases, it is best to normalize the intraocular pressure by removing subretinal fluid, aqueous, or fluid vitreous.

Tonometry is helpful, but of greater interest is the inspection of the central retinal artery. Pulsation of the central retinal artery is clear evidence that blood is definitely entering the retinal circulation. A simple rule of thumb is that the patient may be safely sent to the recovery room if the artery is open at least 50% of the time. The artery is usually fully open by the time the conjunctiva is closed.

If the intraocular pressure is too high, an alternative is to loosen the sutures temporarily. If this is not possible, it is generally advisable to perform paracentesis of the anterior chamber (see Section 6-1-6).

An encircling episcleral buckle can be created with a silicone band. The surgeon

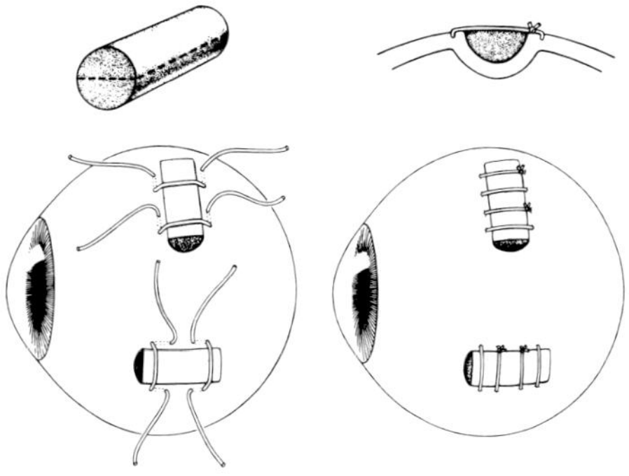

Figure 6-10 *Episcleral buckles with silicone sponge: circumferential and radial.*

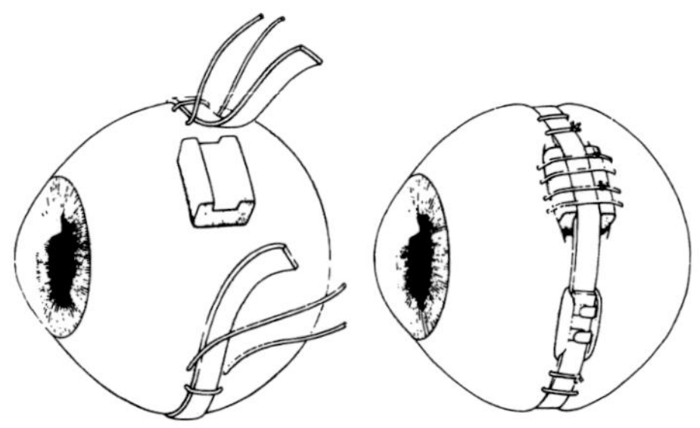

Figure 6-11 *Episcleral buckle with implant and narrow encircling silicone band. Band may be fastened to itself with metal clip, suture, or sleeve. (Compare to Figure 6-9B.)*

may use a narrow band and place appropriate segments of grooved silicone beneath the band where the broader buckle is desired (Figure 6-11). The band is secured to the surface of the globe with mattress sutures.

A surgeon who wants to use only one piece of silicone can select a 4-mm band and position it over the breaks (Figure 6-12). The 4-mm band is sufficiently wide for most breaks, but its effect can be widened at any meridian by the use of supplemental silicone, either sponge or solid. The grooved implant number 280LG (MIRA) has been specifically designed for use with the 4-mm band. The length of the band should be cut to equal the circumference of the patient's globe prior to drainage. If the ends are then overlapped 10 mm, a rather low encircling buckling effect is produced. A moderate buckling effect can be achieved by overlapping 14 mm, and if the surgeon wants a high buckle, as in certain cases of proliferative vitreoretinopathy, the ends are overlapped up to 20 mm.

6-1-5 Drainage of Subretinal Fluid

The drainage of subretinal fluid converts the surgery from an extraocular to an intraocular operation. If drainage is not required, the surgeon can avoid the potential complications of intraocular hemorrhage, iatrogenic retinal break, vitreous loss, retinal incarceration, and intraocular infection. Controversy surrounds the indications for drainage. Some successful surgeons drain almost all cases, while others obtain excellent results by draining infrequently. Most surgeons drain the majority of their cases.

Most surgeons also agree that the surgical drainage of subretinal fluid is indicated for detachments with giant retinal breaks, proliferative vitreoretinopathy, detachments without apparent breaks, and detachments with breaks that do not adequately explain the distribution of subretinal fluid. In addition, many surgeons prefer to drain fluid in cases of posterior retinal tear, high bullous detachment, multiple retinal breaks, aphakia, detachment of the pars plana, and inferior retinal breaks. Many inferior retinal dialyses can be adequately handled without drainage, but inferior breaks near the equator may remain open if the fluid is not drained, because fluid tends to gravitate inferiorly whenever the patient's head is elevated.

There are no universally accepted criteria for drainage. Frequently, the judgment about whether to drain can best be made by the surgeon at the operating table. If the break can be closed at the time of surgery, the fluid elsewhere in the fundus can be left undrained with the expectation of postoperative absorption. If the volume of subretinal fluid during a period of preoperative patching decreases significantly, the surgeon tends to expect that further absorption of the fluid will occur postoperatively even if the break is not completely closed at the time of surgery.

The site for fluid drainage must be carefully selected. Some surgeons prefer to drain underneath the silicone buckle; others favor a site posterior to the buckle. If the former is chosen and if an iatrogenic retinal break or retinal incarceration is inadvertently produced at the drainage site, the surgeon is prepared to immediately support the break or incarceration on the buckle. Drainage is contraindicated in the

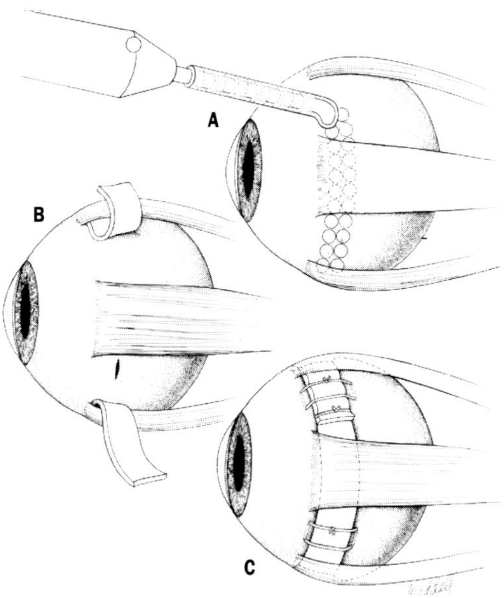

Figure 6-12 *Episcleral buckle with wide encircling band. (A) Cryotherapy. (B) Band length cut to equal circumference of undrained globe, drainage of subretinal fluid. (C) Band tied with 14-mm overlap of cut ends.*

immediate vicinity of the vortex ampullae because of the tendency to create hemorrhage. Therefore, it is preferable to drain near the horizontal recti rather than near the vertical recti. Also, drainage should not be attempted near large retinal breaks, because there may be loss of vitreous through the break. The risk of hemorrhage is greater with a posterior drainage site, because the choroid is more vascular posteriorly. Exposure is much easier on the temporal aspect of the globe, but some surgeons prefer to drain nasally if possible, because any inadvertent subretinal hemorrhage cannot easily reach the macula. The drainage should generally be carried out at a site where the retina is highly elevated. The elevation can be determined immediately before drainage by ophthalmoscopic examination of the retina, with the globe in the position that it will occupy at the moment of choroidal perforation.

The drainage of fluid is usually accomplished near the end of the procedure, when all diathermy or cryotherapy is completed and the silicone buckling material is in place but the buckling sutures are not yet tied securely. Occasionally, it is preferable to drain the subretinal fluid initially and restore the volume with an intravitreal injection of balanced salt solution. Then, with better visualization, the surgeon can proceed with localization, cryotherapy, and buckling. For example, a very bullous detachment in which there is difficulty localizing the retinal break would be a case for initial drainage.

The majority of surgeons prefer to do a drainage sclerotomy with a disposable surgical knife, such as a No. 64 Beaver blade, followed by choroidotomy with the tip of a surgical needle or a needle-shaped diathermy electrode. This is performed while observing the exposed choroid.

Traditionally, the sclerotomy has been radial in orientation and the surgeon or the assistant grasps at least one edge of the scleral wound to expose the choroid. Cautery may be applied to the edges of the sclerotomy to make the wound gape. Another satisfactory alternative is to use a circumferential sclerotomy in which the surgeon grasps the anterior lip. This easily produces gaping of the wound and exposes the choroid. The surgeon is also able to maintain the orientation of the globe with the forceps, and therefore the assistant is not tempted to exert traction on the traction sutures. The surgeon can then easily perform the choroidotomy with the other hand.

The sclerotomy should be 3 to 4 mm in length (Figure 6-13). For an extremely posterior sclerotomy, the surgeon may prefer to use an angled Beaver knife, such as a No. 72. By means of repeated strokes of the knife, the sclera is cut down until the black choroid is exposed. The surface of the choroid should then be carefully examined to avoid the perforation of large choroidal blood vessels. Some surgeons prefer to examine the choroid with a magnifying lens or transillumination. If a choroidal vessel appears within the sclerotomy site, a new sclerotomy should be prepared. Just before the choroidotomy, the surgeon should check to make sure that there is no pressure on the globe from the speculum or from the traction sutures. The choroid should then be perforated by introducing the tip of the drainage needle approximately 2 mm. The needle should be introduced tangentially to minimize the possibility of perforating the retina. A small choroidotomy with controlled drainage is desirable because a large hole in the choroid, with a sudden release of gushing fluid, can create a tendency for the retina to rapidly come against the sclerotomy and produce retinal incarceration or rupture.

As fluid flows into the surgical field, it can be removed by suction or cotton-tipped applicators. If the sclerotomy is covered with silicone, it is not necessary to close the incision with a suture, but the sclerotomy should be closed with a suture if it is not covered by the implant material or if intraocular gas may be used later in the procedure.

6-1-6 Paracentesis of the Anterior Chamber

Scleral buckling without drainage of subretinal fluid, or intravitreal gas injection, may elevate the intraocular pressure enough to occlude the central retinal artery temporarily. The pressure can be lowered with paracentesis of the anterior chamber.

Paracentesis is not recommended in aphakic eyes because of the tendency toward incarceration of a strand of vitreous in the paracentesis site, with peaking of the pupil. Paracentesis is also contraindicated if there is an iris-plane or anterior-chamber intraocular lens, but it is safe

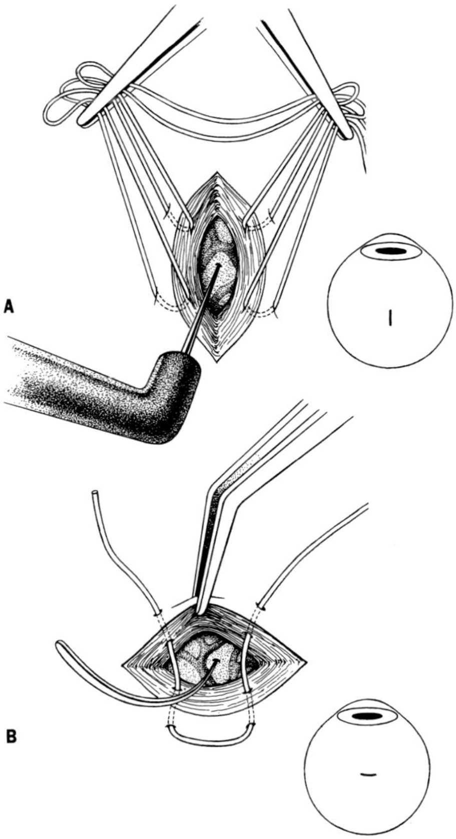

Figure 6-13 *Sclerotomy and choroidotomy for drainage of subretinal fluid, using electrode needle or surgical needle. (A) Radial sclerotomy. (B) Circumferential sclerotomy.*

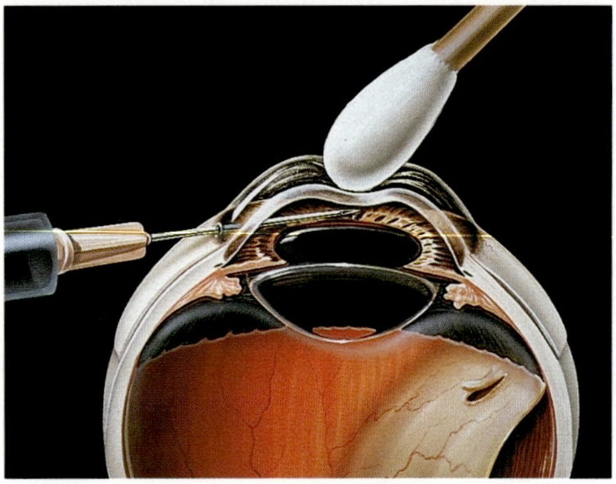

Figure 6-14 *Paracentesis of anterior chamber using 0.5-inch, 30-gauge needle on tuberculin syringe without plunger. Needle is placed between iris and cornea, not in pupil. Central corneal pressure stablizes eye and facilitates complete removal of aqueous humor.*

with a posterior-chamber intraocular lens if the posterior lens capsule is intact or if a small posterior capsulotomy is well covered by the lens. Paracentesis is safely accomplished with a 0.5-inch, 30-gauge needle on a tuberculin syringe without a plunger. It is facilitated by putting pressure on the center of the cornea with a cotton-tipped applicator, which forces fluid toward the chamber angle. The tip of the needle should be placed over the iris near the angle (Figure 6-14).

6-1-7 Intravitreal Injection and Aspiration

The most frequently used vitreous procedure is injection with balanced salt solution, air, or gas. The most common indication for injection is marked hypotony with a partially collapsed globe. Normal intraocular pressure can be restored by injecting balanced salt solution. The injection is made through the pars plana. It is not done anterior to muscle insertions so as to avoid the anterior ciliary arteries. The solution is drawn into a syringe, and all air is carefully eliminated. A 0.5-inch, 30-gauge disposable needle is recommended. As the surgeon grasps the sclera with a twist pic or forceps, the needle is introduced into the vitreous cavity 4 mm posterior to the limbus (Figure 6-15). The tip of the needle is directed toward the geometric center of the globe. In a very soft eye, the tip of the needle may occasionally elevate the pars plana epithelium without perforation. Injection in that situation would produce detachment of the pars plana and retina. This can be avoided by direct visualization of the tip of the needle through the pupil and, when the needle is definitely within the vitreous cavity, the injection can be safely carried out. In phakic eyes, care must be taken to keep the tip of the needle near the middle of the vitreous cavity to avoid touching the lens and subsequent cataract. After injection of the required volume to restore normal intraocular pressure, the needle may be withdrawn. The self-sealing wound does not require suturing.

Another purpose of intravitreal injection is to close a retinal break, especially a gaping break that is aggravated by scleral buckling—the "fish-mouth phenomenon." This is done by pressing the retina outward toward the retinal pigment epithelium. The most popular substance for the injection is air that has been sterilized by passage through a millipore filter. The technique is similar to that described for restoring normal intraocular pressure, except that the needle is inserted at the uppermost aspect of the pars plana and the injection is performed briskly. The air bubble diminishes in volume with time and is usually absorbed within 5 or 6 days.

In an attempt to find a substitute for air that is not so readily absorbed, inert gases—such as sulfur hexafluoride (SF_6) and the fluorocarbon gases (eg, perfluoropropane)—have been introduced. Fluorocarbon gases expand more and persist longer than SF_6, which lasts approximately 10 days. The bubble immediately rises in the vitreous cavity. Therefore, the patient is positioned postoperatively with the retinal break uppermost to provide gas tamponade against the break.

Many detachments with giant breaks are managed with vitrectomy, but some cases (eg, less than 180°) respond well to a low, encircling scleral buckle without vit-

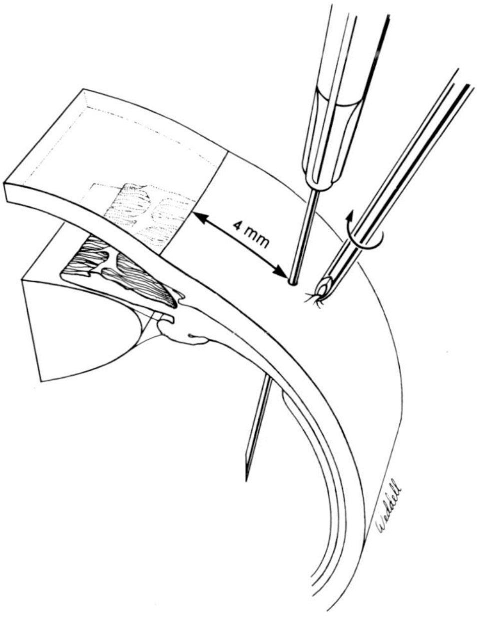

Figure 6-15 *Intravitreal injection through pars plana using twist pic and 30-gauge disposable needle.*

rectomy when the buckle is assisted by the use of a moderate-sized gas bubble. Postoperatively, the patient is managed with appropriate rotating maneuvers to sweep the retina into the desired position as the patient is moved about the bubble (Figure 6-16). The patient is then kept in the desired position postoperatively until the retinal break is sealed.

Aspiration of fluid vitreous through the pars plana is required infrequently. It may be indicated by the need to create space for the placement of a large scleral buckle when it is not necessary to drain subretinal fluid or when the volume of subretinal fluid is very small. Aspiration may also be employed to create intraocular space for the injection of air or gas for the management of a giant retinal break, macular break, or fish-mouth break. Vitreous aspiration can frequently be accomplished by introducing a ⅝-inch, 25-gauge needle 4 mm posterior to the limbus, with the needle tip in the posterior portion of the vitreous cavity. It is helpful to have a very small volume of balanced salt solution in the syringe. When the needle is in place, 0.1-ml solution should be injected. This tends to displace vitreous gel at the tip of the needle and thereby facilitate the aspiration of fluid vitreous. If this is not successful, it is recommended that the surgeon use a 20-gauge needle connected to a 5-ml syringe via a short connecting tube (filled with balanced salt solution). A partial-thickness sclerotomy is made 4 mm posterior to the limbus. The needle is then passed through the vitreous to a position in front of the optic nerve head. This procedure should be carefully monitored by the surgeon with binocular indirect ophthalmoscopy. Fluid vitreous can then be aspirated by the assistant. As the needle is removed, a preplaced absorbable suture is secured to close the sclerotomy. If aspiration does not yield sufficient fluid, the surgeon may resort to the use of a vitrectomy suction-cutter.

6-1-8 Closing the Wound

After placement of the scleral buckle, the excess silicone should be carefully trimmed, especially in very anterior buckles. Tenotomy of extraocular muscles is rarely indicated, but if it is required, the muscle should be resutured to the insertion stump. An absorbable suture, such as 5-0 Dexon, is recommended.

Irrigation of the operative field with an antibiotic solution is strongly advised. Several different types of antibiotics have been used successfully, such as a combination of neomycin, gramicidin, and polymyxin B (Neosporin Ophthalmic Solution) or cephazolin (Ancef). Approximately 10 ml is drawn into a syringe, and the field is then irrigated using a blunt-tipped needle. The irrigation should be deep in the plane between Tenon's capsule and the sclera in all opened quadrants. Before any implant material is used, it should be soaked in the same antibiotic solution.

If the conjunctival incision was posterior to the limbus, the wound may be

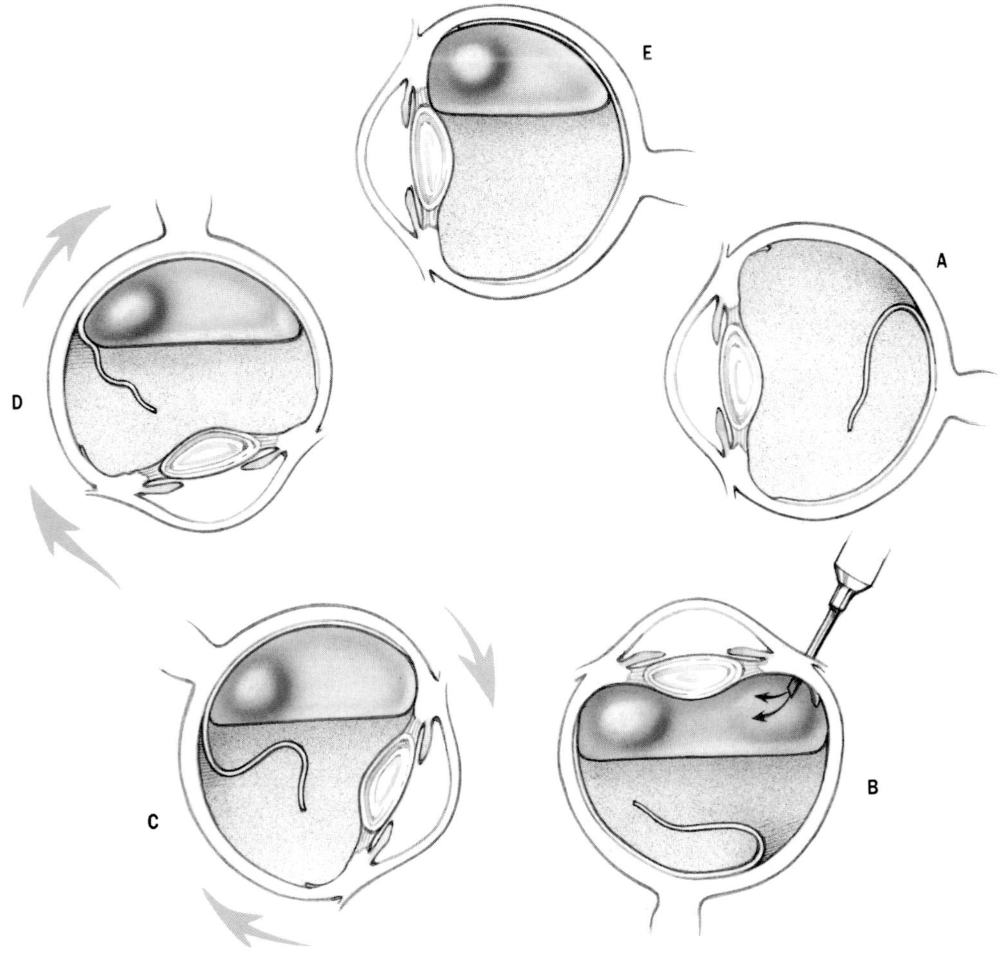

Figure 6-16 *Gas injection and manipulation of retinal flap by bubble for superior giant tear with rolled-over flap. (A) Preoperative tear. (B) Injection of 2.5 ml of 20% SF_6 (80% sterile air). (C) Movement of bubble to inferior fundus during backward somersault (few hours postoperative). (D) Continuation of somersault positions; bubble at posterior pole. (E) Final postoperative position.*

Redrawn with permission from Rice TA, Michels RG, Stark WJ, eds: Ophthalmic Surgery. *4th ed. London: Butterworth & Co, Ltd; 1984.*

closed with a 5-0 plain catgut running suture, 360°. With such an incision, most surgeons elect to close Tenon's capsule first with several interrupted sutures, before closing the conjunctiva with the running suture. If the initial incision was at the limbus, it is not necessary to close Tenon's capsule separately; both Tenon's capsule and the conjunctiva may be closed together. Limbal peritomy is usually associated with two relaxing incisions perpendicular to the limbus. Each can be closed with one or two interrupted sutures. Some postoperative suture discomfort can be eliminated by burying the suture knots in Tenon's space.

The normal tendency for postoperative chemosis is aggravated if conjunctiva is left over the surface of the cornea at the end of the procedure. If a limbal peritomy was performed, care should be taken to keep the conjunctiva 2 or 3 mm posterior to the limbus. The use of a moderate pressure dressing also helps to minimize chemosis. Dressing only the operated eye is usually sufficient. Bilateral bandages may be considered in a nondrainage operation if the break is still open.

6-1-9 Reoperations

In different series, 5% to 15% of retinal detachments have required two or more operations to effect a permanent reattachment. Such procedures are indicated by persistence of the initial detachment or recurrence of the detachment.

Meticulous examination is required to identify the leaking retinal breaks. Attention is often directed to the posterior edge of the original break, but it should be remembered that some failures are due to leakage of the fluid anterior to the buckle. Fluid may dissect inferiorly and then present over an encircling buckle in the inferior part of the fundus. The distribution of the subretinal fluid should be carefully recorded on the fundus drawing, and the dictum that "water runs downhill" is usually a guide to the most likely area of the leaking break.

In the case of an encircling scleral buckle, if all the fluid is posterior to the buckle, the break must certainly be behind the buckle. However, if the subretinal fluid passes anterior to the buckle in one area, that is the most likely site for the leaking break.

The most difficult part of the reoperation is opening. The problem ranges from just a nuisance in recently operated cases to a frank hazard in certain old cases that have considerable scarring associated with thin sclera. In a recently operated case (less than 10 days), the surgeon may simply open the conjunctival incision with blunt dissection. Bleeding is usually significant, and therefore suction should be available at the operating table. After several weeks, however, there is considerable scar tissue, and careful sharp dissection is required to identify the plane of the sclera and to elevate Tenon's capsule and the conjunctiva.

It is frequently difficult to pass a muscle hook beneath muscles during a reoperation. If the silicone buckle passes beneath the muscle, it is recommended that the surgeon first approach that buckle with sharp dissection in the middle of the quadrant. The dissection can then be carried along the surface of the silicone until the edge of the muscle is reached. The muscle hook can be passed along the surface of the silicone beneath the muscle, which enables passage of a traction suture beneath the muscle.

Occasionally, there is so much scar tissue around the muscle that repeated attempts to pass a muscle hook should be abandoned. A traction suture on a scleral needle can simply be passed through the sclera anterior to the muscle insertion. However, if the reoperation requires the placement of buckling material beneath the muscle, it should be temporarily tenotomized and carefully dissected free from the surface of the sclera.

The process of opening is relatively easy after episcleral buckles with cryotherapy. However, if there has been surface diathermy, greater care is required because Tenon's capsule is adherent to the sclera and diathermy can weaken the sclera.

Occasionally, an area of very thin sclera is encountered, and if the globe is ruptured or if rupture is imminent, steps should be taken to strengthen the area. In small scleral dehiscences, the surgeon may simply imbricate the sclera at that point, but larger defects may require the placement of donor sclera as a patch. Donor sclera can be preserved for many years in 95% ethyl alcohol, and when required it can be readily prepared for use by three successive baths (6 minutes each) in normal saline solution. It is well to keep such sclera on hand in the operating room. The scleral patch may be secured with sutures or with cyanoacrylate glue.

After the painstaking process of opening has been completed, the surgeon may perform the required treatment. The use of diathermy requires careful dissection down to the plane of the sclera and is preferably applied through thinned sclera under scleral flaps. This difficult procedure can be avoided by the use of cryotherapy, which can be applied through sclera of varying thicknesses and even through episcleral scar tissue. Each application should be monitored by ophthalmoscopy. Additional scleral buckling can be done with episcleral silicone. When this technique is used, the surgeon need not dissect down through episcleral scar to expose an extensive area of bare sclera, but is required only to expose the sclera in those sites where the suture needle will be passed through it. Cryotherapy should be applied around the area of the retinal breaks, but if there is considerable atrophy of the choroid and pigment epithelium, additional cryotherapy should be applied widely around the break into adjacent areas of normal choroid.

Drainage is frequently indicated in a reoperation. This procedure is complicated by the fact that the choroid may be somewhat engorged. The surgeon may require a slightly larger drainage needle to create an adequate opening in the thickened choroid.

Redundance of episcleral tissues is often encountered in a reoperation. All devitalized tissue should be carefully debrided to minimize the increased risk of infection

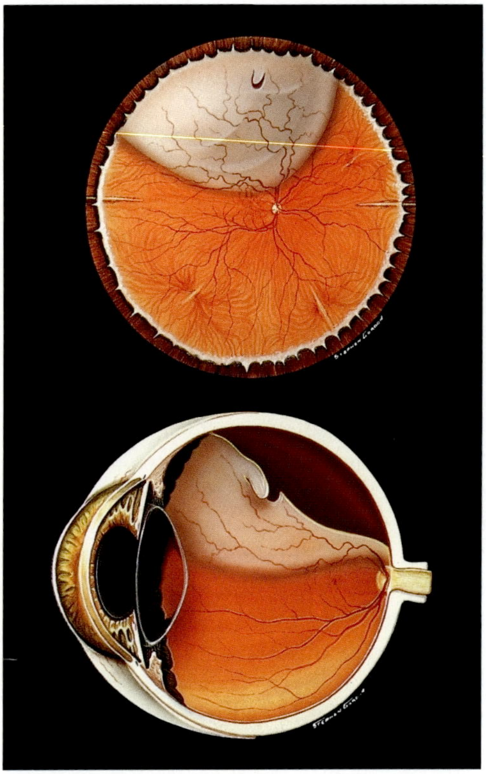

Figure 6-17 *Quadrantic detachment with one break.*

that is associated with reoperation. The surgical wound should be copiously irrigated with an antibiotic solution before closing. Most detachments can be managed with only one or two reoperations, but in rare instances as many as four or five have been required to achieve a cure. The indications for such persistence depend on the individual case.

6-1-10 Twelve Representative Cases

Most retinal detachments can be cured with one of several different techniques. There is no one right way. The choice of procedure is influenced by each surgeon's background and training. Some surgical techniques are discussed below, but they are not the only approaches. In this section, cryotherapy is described, but in each case diathermy could be used instead.

6-1-10-1 Quadrantic Detachment With One Break A quadrantic detachment with only one break can be managed with several applications of contiguous cryotherapy surrounding the break (Figure 6-17). The posterior limit of the retinal break is localized on the surface of the sclera. A silicone sponge is sutured to the surface of the globe, creating a segmental scleral buckle. Drainage of subretinal fluid is not usually necessary, but if the break remains widely open after buckling, the surgeon may release the fluid by untying the sutures to restore normal intraocular pressure and then draining the fluid. An alternative is the trap-door procedure, in which scleral flaps are dissected and silicone or gelatin is placed to produce an intrascleral buckle. If the break is located in the superior two thirds of the fundus, pneumatic retinopexy may also be considered (see Section 6-2-3).

6-1-10-2 Total Detachment With One Break The most common location for a break in total detachment is near the 12-o'clock meridian (Figure 6-18). If there are no other suspicious areas and if the fundus can be thoroughly examined, the surgeon can simply use cryotherapy and place a segmental silicone sponge at the site of the break. Most surgeons prefer to drain subretinal fluid, but many cases have been managed satisfactorily without drainage. However, an encircling procedure should be performed if any of the following conditions is present:

1. The retinal break is not in the expected position.
2. There is some question as to the integrity of the peripheral retina.
3. There is any evidence of proliferative vitreoretinopathy.
4. The peripheral retina cannot be fully examined in all areas.

Pneumatic retinopexy might also be considered if the break is located in the superior two thirds of the fundus: clockwise from 8 to 4 o'clock (see Section 6-2-3).

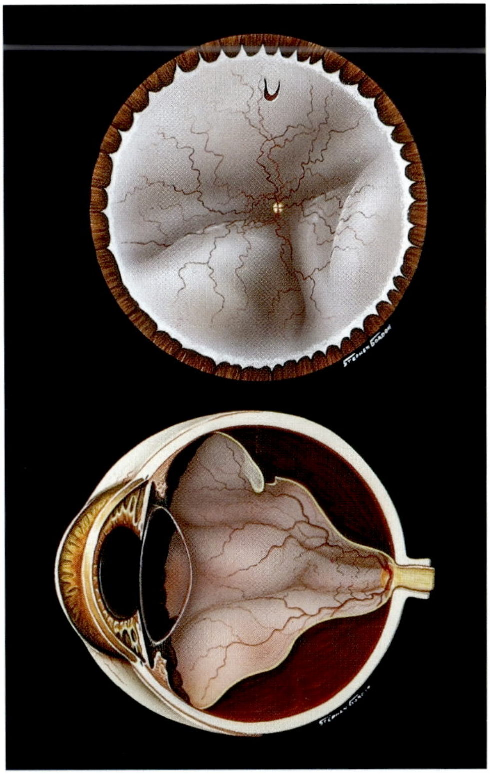

Figure 6-18 *Total detachment with one break.*

6-1-10-3 Detachment With Multiple Breaks at Same Distance From Ora An encircling buckle is recommended for a detachment with multiple breaks at the same distance from the ora serrata (Figure 6-19). If the breaks are of average size, they can be adequately managed with a 4-mm silicone band without any additional silicone implants. How-

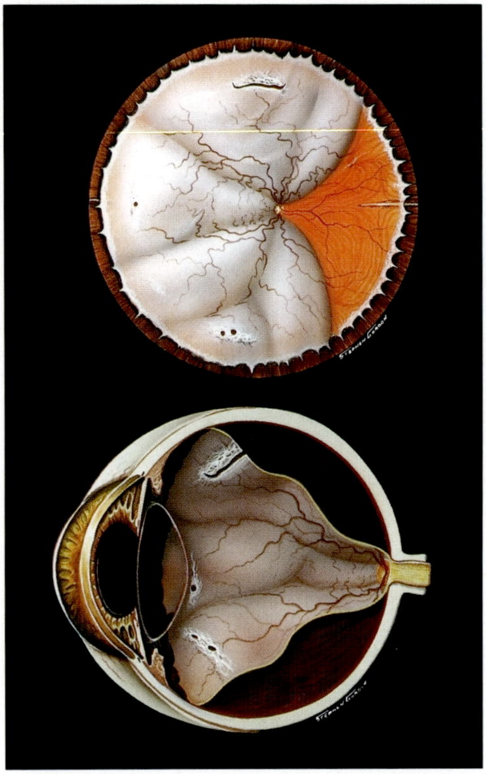

Figure 6-19 *Detachment with multiple breaks at same distance from ora.*

ever, if one or more of the breaks are larger than average, the surgeon should supplement the buckle with a wider piece of silicone placed beneath the band. Each break should be surrounded with cryotherapy and localized on the sclera. The sutures should then be oriented so as to place the breaks on the crest of the buckle. Subretinal fluid may be drained. Alternatively, the surgeon might use a narrow band and place a grooved implant beneath the band to support the breaks.

6-1-10-4 Detachment With Multiple Breaks at Different Distances From Ora In detachment with multiple breaks at different distances from the ora serrata, each of the breaks should be treated with cryotherapy (Figure 6-20). Then a broad, grooved silicone implant, called a *tire*, can be employed to place all the breaks on a broad buckle. The implant is usually used in association with an encircling band. It is sutured to the surface of the globe for a cryotherapy procedure, but if diathermy is selected, the surgeon should dissect scleral flaps. Subretinal fluid is usually drained. Another approach to this problem is to use a wide silicone sponge, 7.5 to 12 mm, in a circumferential orientation to create a wide buckle.

6-1-10-5 "Aphakic Detachment" With Multiple Small Ora Breaks In an aphakic detachment with multiple small ora breaks, each of the breaks should be treated with cryotherapy (Figure 6-21). An encircling buckle is recommended, and it should be placed immediately posterior to the ora breaks. Drainage of subretinal fluid is usually required.

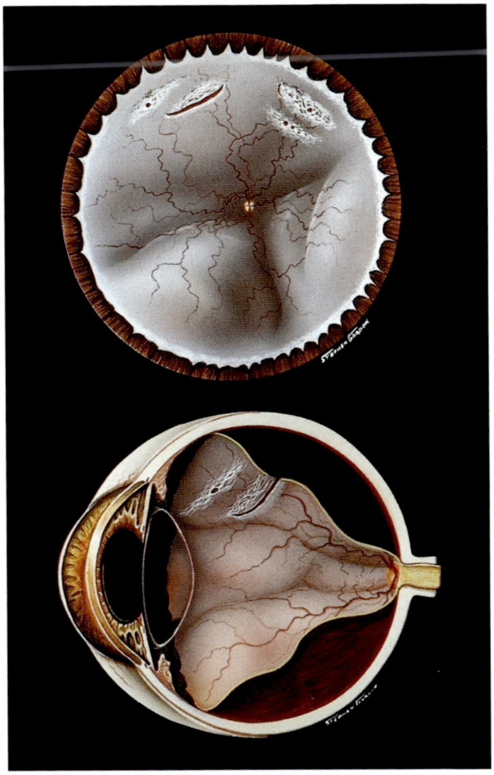

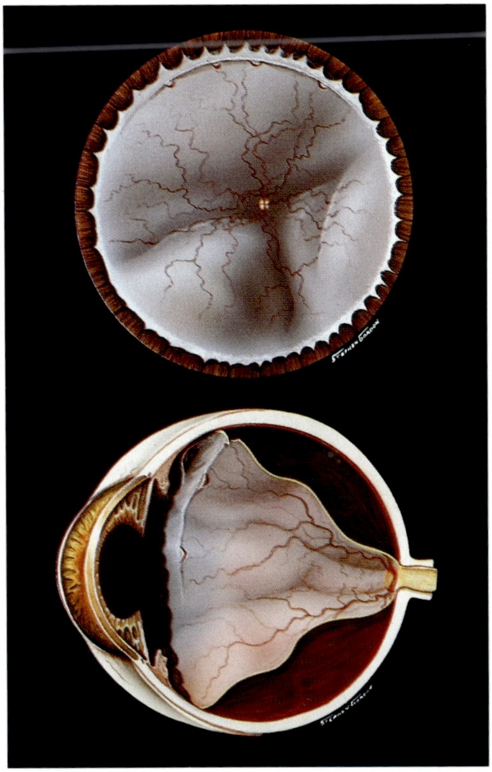

6-1-10-6 Detachment With Peripheral Break and Macular Hole A detachment with a peripheral break and a macular hole is generally managed with cryotherapy and buckling of the peripheral break with no treatment to the apparent macular hole (Figure 6-22). Macular holes are usually secondary cystic changes and are not causally related to the rhegmatogenous retinal detachment. If, however, fluid reaccumulates around the posterior hole in the early postoperative course, a second procedure—usually pneumatic retinopexy—is required to close the hole.

Figure 6-20 *(Left) Detachment with multiple breaks at different distances from ora.*

Figure 6-21 *(Right) "Aphakic detachment" with multiple small ora breaks.*

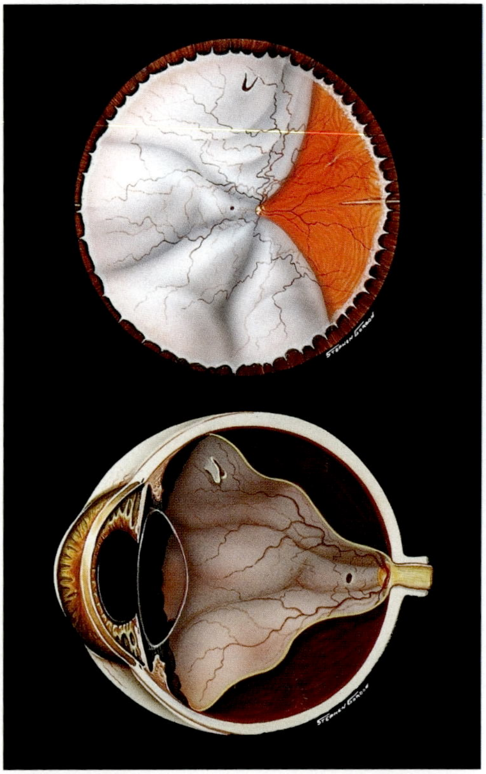

Figure 6-22 *Detachment with peripheral break and macular hole.*

6-1-10-7 Detachment due to Macular Break Detachments caused by macular breaks are generally seen in association with high myopia, which is frequently accompanied by posterior staphyloma, or in cases of ocular trauma (Figure 6-23). These breaks are often difficult to visualize. They may be small and irregular or slit-like in configuration, and are usually not located in the center of the foveola but somewhat eccentrically. Pneumatic retinopexy is recommended (see Section 6-2-3). Gas is injected into the vitreous. After 1 day of face-down positioning of the patient, the retina will usually be reattached and the break may be treated with extrafoveolar laser photocoagulation. If this fails, vitrectomy with fluid–gas exchange may be considered. If that also fails, the surgeon might use a scleral buckle at the macula, but this is very rarely required. The surgeon creates a buckle in the form of the letter Y with a 3×5-mm sponge, the ends of which are sutured near the equator in three quadrants. Alternatively, an implant may be sutured to the sclera of the posterior pole. Drainage of subretinal fluid is usually required.

6-1-10-8 Detachment With Retinal Dialysis A detachment with a retinal dialysis is seen most often in juveniles or young adults and is referred to as the inferior dialysis of the young syndrome (Figure 6-24). However, dialyses may occur in any quadrant at any age. The posterior margin of the dialysis should be treated with contiguous cryotherapy and by securing a segmental episcleral sponge buckle to the surface of the globe with several mattress sutures. The buckle should be placed just behind

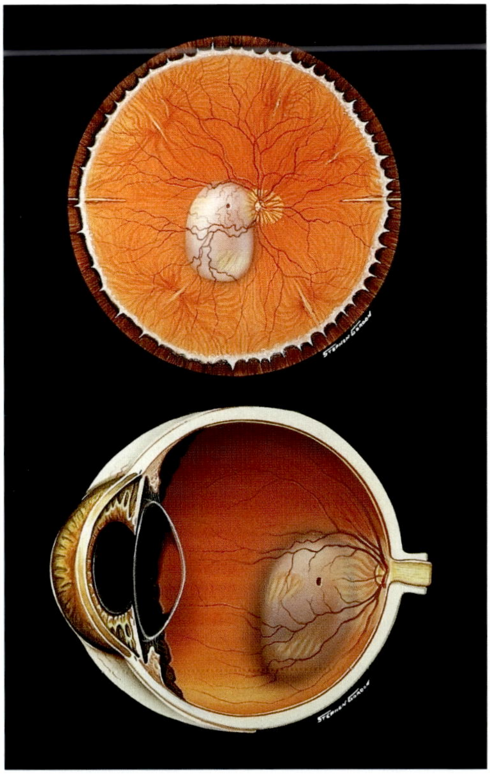

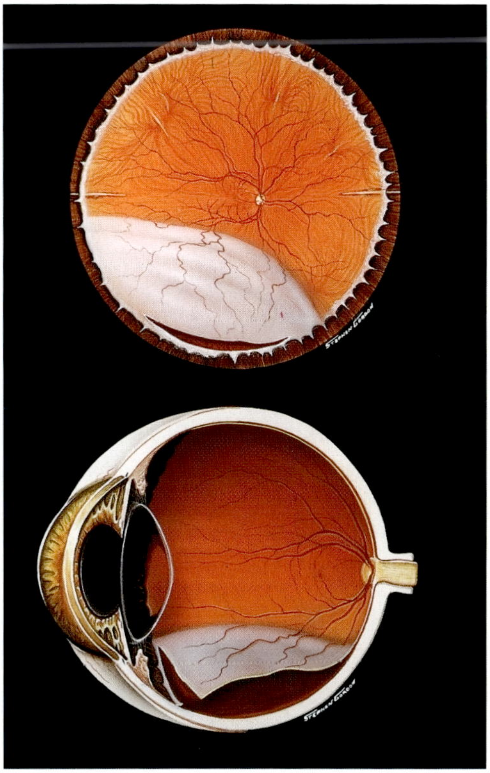

Figure 6-23 *(Left) Detachment due to macular break.*

Figure 6-24 *(Right) Detachment with retinal dialysis.*

the posterior edge of the break. Drainage of subretinal fluid is optional. Buckling with scleral infolding or absorbable gelatin also yields good results and eliminates the need for a permanent implant.

6-1-10-9 Detachment With Giant Break A giant break is generally defined as a break of 90° or more (Figure 6-25). In the case of a giant break with a rolled-over flap, its entire edge and the area posterior to the break are treated with multiple applications of contiguous cryotherapy. A rather low encircling scleral buckle is employed. Subretinal fluid is drained. If adequate

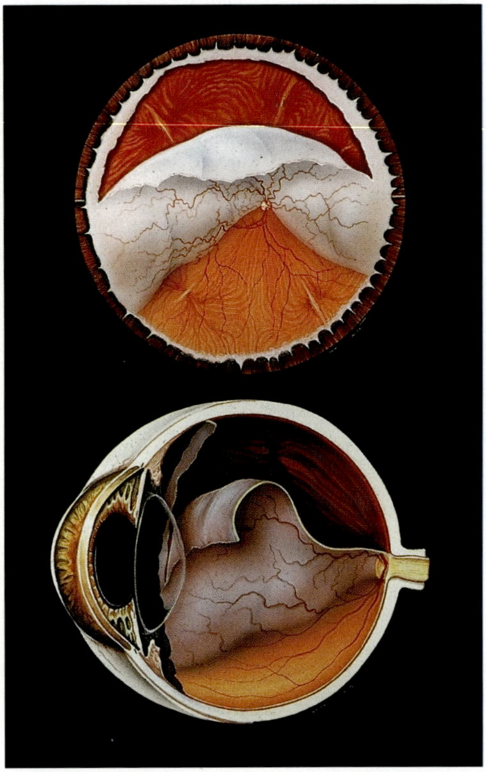

Figure 6-25 *Detachment with giant break.*

fluid cannot be obtained, the surgeon may have to aspirate fluid vitreous and perhaps also do a paracentesis of the anterior chamber. After drainage, a nonexpansile intravitreal bubble of gas, such as 20% SF_6, should be injected so that it occupies approximately half the vitreous cavity. Postoperatively, the patient is manipulated with a rotating maneuver to roll the bubble across the retina and sweep the flap into the proper position. The patient then maintains the appropriate posture until the break is sealed, which may require 5 to 10 days of critical postoperative positioning (see Figure 6-16). Vitrectomy, including the use of heavier-than-water perfluorocarbon liquid, is recommended for rolled-over breaks that exceed 180°, for recurrences, and especially for breaks with associated proliferative vitreoretinopathy.

6-1-10-10 Detachment With No Apparent Break The difficult problem of a detachment with no apparent break is best managed by the application of two rows of contiguous cryotherapy just posterior to the ora in all detached quadrants (Figure 6-26). Subretinal fluid should be drained, and an encircling 4-mm scleral buckle placed between the ora and the equator (see Figure 6-12). Surgery should not be performed until secondary detachment (due to uveitis, tumor, or other entities) has been carefully ruled out.

6-1-10-11 Detachment With Outer-Layer Break in Retinoschisis Minimal subretinal fluid requires no treatment. Moderate subretinal fluid (2 to 4 disc diameters) may frequently be managed with cryotherapy or photocoagulation. But if there is a clinical

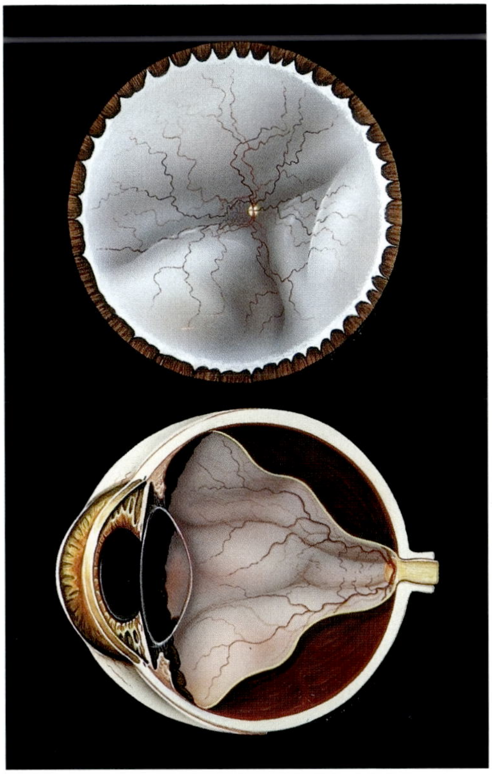

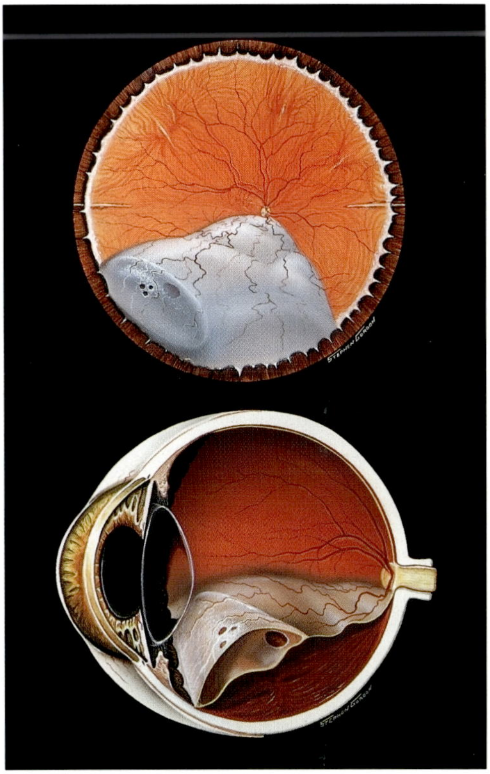

retinal detachment, each of the outer-layer breaks should be carefully treated with cryotherapy and closed with scleral buckling (Figure 6-27). Subretinal fluid can be drained as indicated. These maneuvers generally cure the retinal detachment. If the surgeon also wants to collapse the retinoschisis cavity, additional cryotherapy should be applied to cover the entire retinoschisis area. With such cryotherapy, the retinoschisis cavity partially collapses after several weeks, and occasionally totally collapses. Inner-layer breaks require no treatment and can safely be ignored.

Figure 6-26 *(Left) Detachment with no apparent break.*

Figure 6-27 *(Right) Detachment with outer-layer break in retinoschisis.*

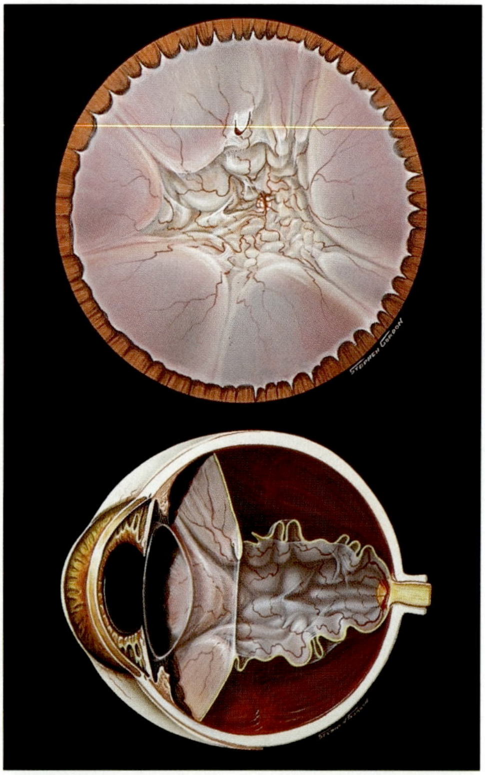

Figure 6-28 *Detachment with proliferative vitreoretinopathy, Grade D-2.*

6-1-10-12 Detachment With Proliferative Vitreoretinopathy This most difficult problem, detachment with proliferative vitreoretinopathy, has a limited prognosis (Figure 6-28). Grade C-1 or C-2 (see Table 3-3) can frequently be cured with a high encircling buckle. For Grade C-3 or greater, vitrectomy techniques are recommended.

6-2

ALTERNATIVE PROCEDURES

Although scleral buckling with permanent implants has been the standard treatment of retinal detachment for many years, several alternative procedures have been successfully utilized.

6-2-1 Photocoagulation

Photocoagulation of the retina, without scleral buckling or gas, can occasionally be utilized for a very small retinal detachment, measuring approximately 2 to 4 disc diameters. This has been accomplished with the xenon-arc photocoagulator or the slip-lamp laser, but the preferred technique at this time is the laser indirect ophthalmoscope with scleral indentation. The latter method ensures adequate photocoagulation on the anterior margin of the break, and the treatment can be easily extended out to the ora serrata. This method usually delimits the small detachment and occasionally also totally flattens the retina. The reason for such flattening is not well understood, but it has been conjectured that this treatment may produce a fibrin coagulum at the break site and somewhat reduce the inflow of fluid vitreous, thereby allowing the retinal pigment epithelial pump to remove all subretinal fluid.

6-2-2 Cryotherapy

Transconjunctival cryotherapy of the retina has the same indications as described above for photocoagulation. But the cryotherapy technique is generally utilized if the media are not clear enough for photocoagulation, but clear enough to visualize the retinal breaks.

6-2-3 Pneumatic Retinopexy

The basic indications for pneumatic retinopexy are:

1. The break (or cluster of breaks) is no larger than the 1-o'clock hour.

2. The break is located superiorly between 8 and 4 o'clock.

3. There is no proliferative vitreoretinopathy greater than Grade C-1.

Special indications include detachments with: optic pit, macular break, very posterior or irregular breaks, filtering bleb, very thin sclera, very scarred conjunctiva, the need to maintain emmetropia, and the need to prevent cosmetic problems such as ptosis, enophthalmos, or strabismus.

Pneumatic retinopexy consists of transconjunctival cryotherapy, intravitreal gas injection, and postoperative positioning to close the retinal break with the gas bubble. The break is treated with multiple contiguous applications of cryotherapy, while monitoring by binocular indirect ophthalmoscopy. The use of an eyelid speculum is optional during cryotherapy but is required during gas injection. The cornea and conjunctiva are treated with several drops of topical povidone iodine (Betadine Solution). Other preparations of Betadine contain detergents or alcohol and may injure the cornea, but Betadine Solution is a safe and effective antiseptic. The gas injection is usually made through the pars plana 4 mm posterior to the limbus (Figure 6-29). Perfluorocarbon gases have been used, but sulfur hexafluoride (SF_6) is the most popular. Postoperatively, the patient is instructed to position the head so that the retinal break is uppermost for at least 16 hours a day for 5 days (Figure 6-30).

Occasionally, it is preferable to use a two-session method. If the break is too posterior to be reached with the cryoprobe in the conjunctival cul-de-sac or if the detachment is too bullous to allow accurate placement of cryotherapy, it is preferable only to inject gas at the first session. Then, 1 or 2 days later, after the retina has been pneumatically reattached, the retinal break is treated with cryotherapy or laser photocoagulation. A multicenter randomized controlled clinical trial compared pneumatic retinopexy with traditional scleral buckling. Despite a higher frequency of new or missed retinal breaks, the pneumatic retinopexy group had similar anatomic results, less morbidity, and,

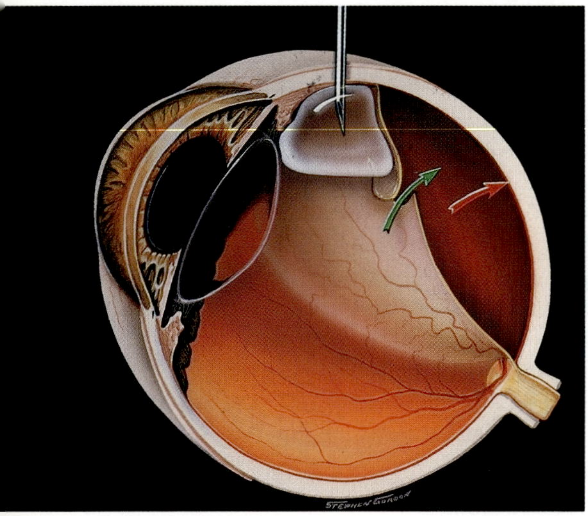

Figure 6-29 *Pneumatic retinopexy. With pars plana injection site uppermost, gas bubble of 0.3 to 0.5 ml is briskly injected into vitreous with 0.5-inch, 30-gauge needle. Only tip of needle is in vitreous cavity.*

Published with permission from Hilton GF, Grizzard WS: Pneumatic retinopexy: a two-step outpatient operation without conjunctival incision. Ophthalmology *1986;93:626–641.*

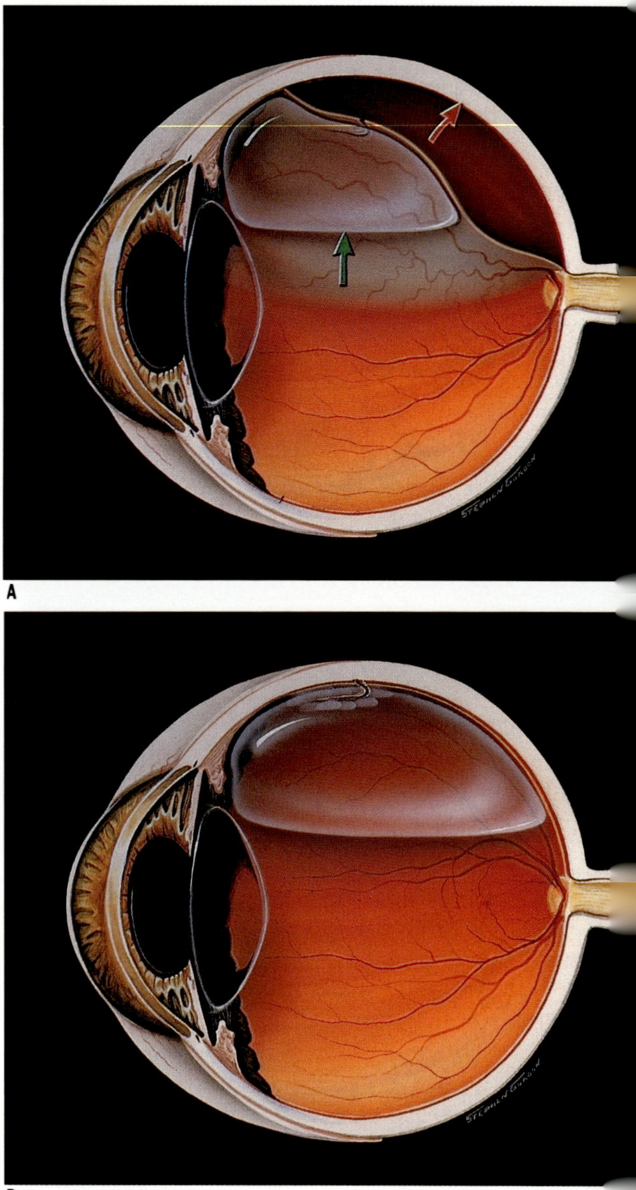

A

B

Figure 6-30 *Pneumatic retinopexy. (A) Patient's head is positioned so as to place retinal break uppermost, thereby sealing break with intravitreal gas bubble. (B) With break closed, retina is usually reattached by first postoperative day.*

Published with permission from Hilton GF, Grizzard WS: Pneumatic retinopexy: a two-step outpatient operation without conjunctival incision. Ophthalmology *1986;93:626–641.*

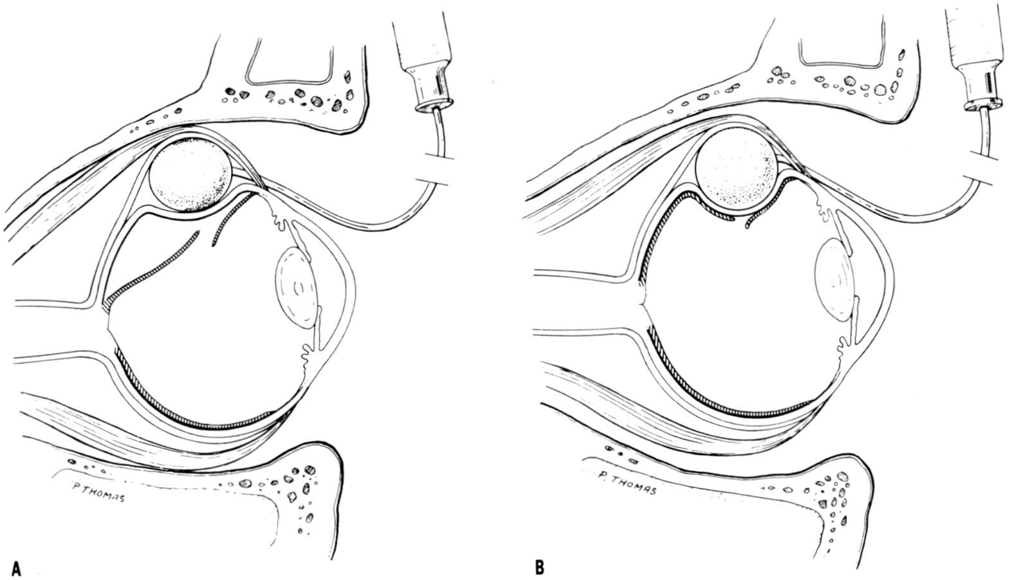

most importantly, better postoperative visual acuity. It has been suggested that treatment of the break after it has been reattached may reduce the incidence of postoperative proliferative vitreoretinopathy (the current incidence is 3% to 4%).

6-2-4 Orbital Balloon

In the orbital balloon procedure, the retinal break is treated with transconjunctival cryotherapy, a deflated balloon is inserted through an incision in the conjunctiva and Tenon's capsule, and the balloon is positioned adjacent to the globe at the retinal break site (Figure 6-31). As the balloon is inflated, the fundus is monitored with binocular indirect ophthalmoscopy. The balloon catheter is temporarily attached to the patient's forehead, and the balloon is left in place for 1 week. The procedure was initially performed on an inpatient ba-

Figure 6-31 *Orbital balloon procedure. (A) Sagittal section of orbit, showing balloon in Tenon's space shortly after insertion. Balloon is compressed between eye and bony orbit. (B) Postoperatively, balloon has closed retinal break, and retina has been reattached.*

Reproduced from Lincoff H, Kreissig I: Results with a temporary balloon buckle for the repair of retinal detachment. Am J Ophthalmol *1981;92:245–251. Published with permission from The American Journal of Ophthalmology. Copyright by The Ophthalmic Publishing Company.*

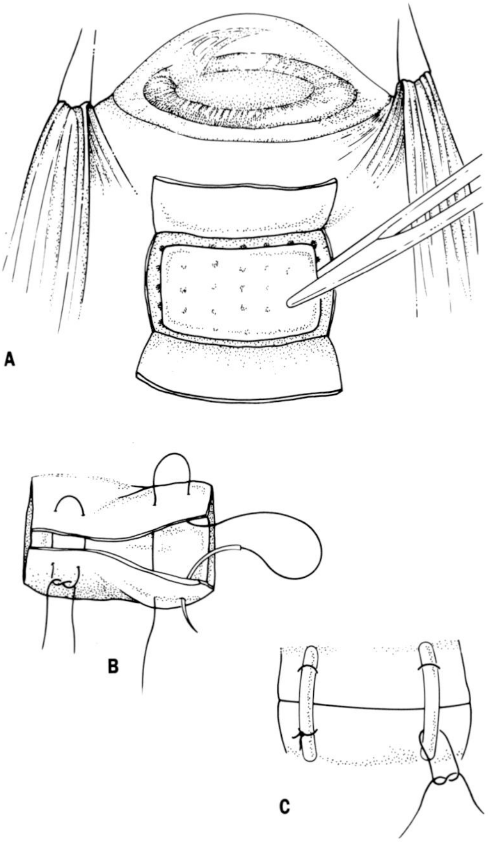

Figure 6-32 *Gelatin scleral buckle. (A) Gelatin implant is trimmed smaller than scleral pocket to permit adequate buckling. (B) Nonabsorbable 4-0 sutures are passed through scleral flaps; 3-0 plain gut under mattress sutures serves as reinforcement. (C) Completed operation.* *Reproduced with permission from Ryan SJ, ed:* Retina. *2nd ed. St Louis: CV Mosby Co; 1994.*

sis, but outpatient use has also yielded good results. After 1 week, the balloon is deflated and removed. Failures usually respond to a permanent scleral buckle.

6-2-5 Gelatin Scleral Buckle

Unless a permanent buckle is absolutely necessary, many surgeons prefer to use a temporary buckle for the treatment of children. One popular method is the placement of gelatin in an intrascleral trap-door procedure (Figure 6-32; see also Figure 6-9). The gelatin may also be simply sutured to the surface of the sclera without the dissection of scleral flaps. Such buckles generally last from 2 to 3 months. If thick blocks of gelatin are not readily available, several sheets of commercially available Gelfilm may be used. Alternatively, a softened sheet of Gelfilm can be rolled into a cylindrical configuration. This procedure is accomplished by soaking the Gelfilm in balanced salt solution until it becomes slightly soft. The gelatin buckle has been used satisfactorily for a number of children with inferior temporal dialyses.

6-3

VITRECTOMY

There have been a few reports on the use of vitrectomy, internal drainage of subretinal fluid, and total fluid–gas exchange without scleral buckling for primary detachments (Figure 6-33). In general, satisfactory results have been obtained, but almost all eyes develop postoperative cataract. Therefore, advocates of this modality

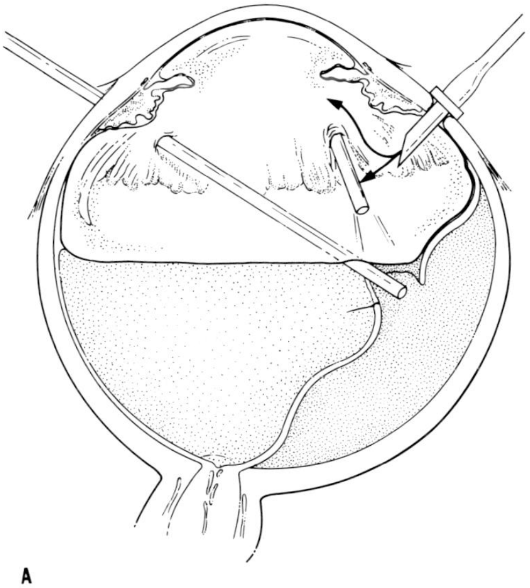

A

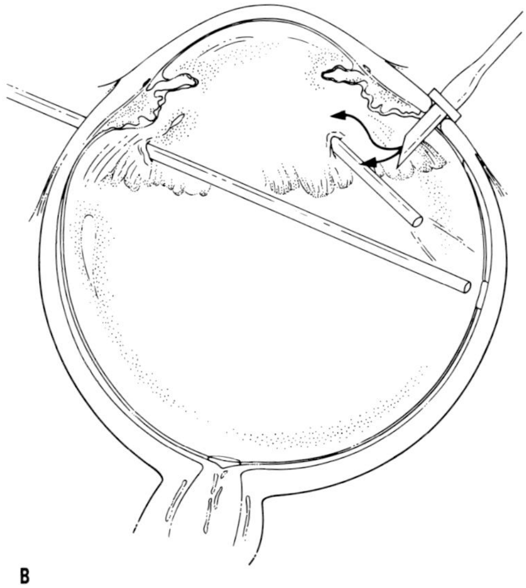

B

Figure 6-33 *Vitrectomy without scleral buckling. (A) After vitrectomy, subretinal fluid is drained internally as fluid–gas exchange is performed. (B) Pneumatic retinal reattachment without scleral buckling.*

Reproduced with permission from Ryan SJ, ed: Retina. *2nd ed. St Louis: CV Mosby Co; 1994.*

now recommend it only for aphakic or pseudophakic detachments.

Some very complicated detachments may require the multiple procedures employed in *vitrectomy* (Figure 6-34), a term originally coined for the surgical excision of the vitreous but now often used for any intraocular microsurgical technique used in the posterior segment. These techniques include pars plana lensectomy, iridectomy, iridotomy, vitrectomy per se, epiretinal membrane segmentation or removal, retinotomy, retinectomy, internal drainage of subretinal fluid, pneumatic retinal reattachment, intravitreal gas or silicone oil, perfluorocarbon liquid, endodiathermy, endocryotherapy, endolaser photocoagulation, retinal suturing, and tissue glue. These elaborate microsurgical techniques have facilitated reattachment of the retina in many cases that would previously have been diagnosed as inoperable.

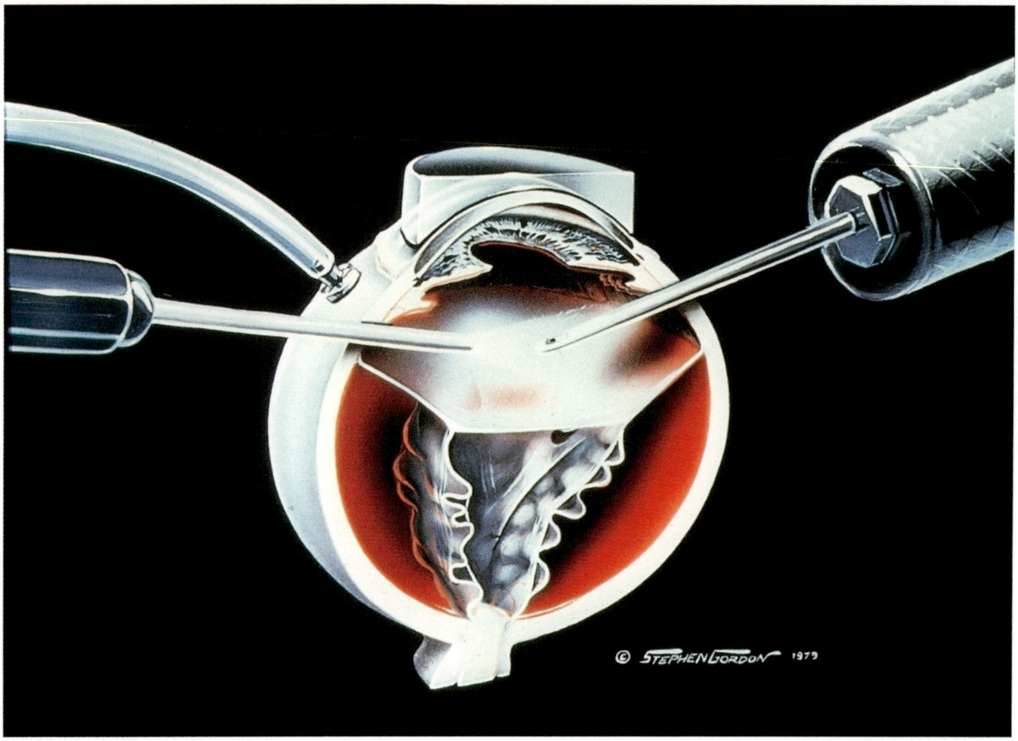

Figure 6-34 *Vitrectomy for aphakic detachment with Grade D-2 proliferative vitreoretinopathy, utilizing three pars plana sclerotomies for suction-cutter, endoilluminator, and infusion cannula.*

Vitrectomy, which would be better termed "microsurgery of the posterior segment," may be considered for retinal detachments with proliferative vitreoretinopathy, detachments with giant breaks, diabetic tractional detachments, any detachments with opacification of the lens or vitreous, and detachments associated with certain types of trauma, including intraocular foreign bodies. Microsurgery of the posterior segment is also useful for the removal of epiretinal membranes in the macula, termed *macular pucker*, which occur after surgical reattachment of the retina in approximately 2% of cases.

SUGGESTED READINGS

American Academy of Ophthalmology: The repair of rhegmatogenous retinal detachment. Information Statement. *Ophthalmology* 1990;97: 1562–1572.

Barricks ME, Shafer DM, Hilton GF: A technique for improving corneal clarity during retinal surgery. *Am J Ophthalmol* 1978;86:274–275.

Escoffery RF, Olk RJ, Grand MG, et al: Vitrectomy without scleral buckling for primary rhegmatogenous retinal detachment. *Am J Ophthalmol* 1985;99:275–281.

Faris B, Freeman HM, Schepens CL: Scleral dehiscences, anterior staphyloma, and retinal detachment, I: incidence and pathogenesis. *Trans Am Acad Ophthalmol Otolaryngol* 1975; 79:OP851–853.

Grand MG: Electrocoaptation conjunctival closure in retinal detachment surgery. *Arch Ophthalmol* 1980;98:1439–1440.

Griffith RD, Ryan EA, Hilton GF: Primary retinal detachments without apparent breaks. *Am J Ophthalmol* 1976;81:420–427.

Grizzard WS, Hilton GF: Scleral buckling for retinal detachments complicated by periretinal proliferation. *Arch Ophthalmol* 1982;100: 419–422.

Hilton GF, Grizzard WS: Pneumatic retinopexy: a two-step outpatient operation without conjunctival incision. *Ophthalmology* 1986; 93:626–641.

Hilton, GF, Grizzard WS, Avins LR, et al: The drainage of subretinal fluid: a randomized controlled clinical trial. *Retina* 1981;1:271–280.

Hilton GF, Kelly NE, Salzano TC, et al: Pneumatic retinopexy: a collaborative report of the first 100 cases. *Ophthalmology* 1987;94: 307–314.

Johnston GP, Okun E, Boniuk I, et al: Drainage of subretinal fluid: why, when, where and how? *Mod Probl Ophthalmol* 1975;15:197–206.

King LM Jr, Margherio RR, Schepens CL: Gelatin implants in scleral buckling procedures. *Arch Ophthalmol* 1975;93:807–811.

King LM Jr, Schepens CL: Limbal peritomy in retinal detachment surgery. *Arch Ophthalmol* 1974;91:295–298.

Kloti R: Retinal detachment surgery without scleral buckling: primary vitrectomy. *Klin Monatsbl Augenheilkd* 1983;182:474–478.

Lincoff H, Coleman J, Kreissig I, et al: The perfluorocarbon gases in the treatment of retinal detachment. *Ophthalmology* 1983;90: 546–551.

Lincoff H, Kreissig I: Advantages of radial buckling. *Am J Ophthalmol* 1975;79:955–957.

Lincoff H, Kreissig I, Richard G, et al: A multicenter trial of the balloon buckle. *Int Congr Ophthalmol* 1982;1:517–519.

Lincoff HA, McLean JM, Nano H: Cryosurgical treatment of retinal detachment. *Trans Am Acad Ophthalmol Otolargyngol* 1964;68:412–432.

McLean EB, Norton EWD: Use of intraocular air and sulfur hexafluoride gas in the repair of selected retinal detachments. *Mod Probl Ophthalmol* 1974;12:428–435.

Michels RG: Scleral buckling methods for rhegmatogenous retinal detachment. *Retina* 1986;6:1–49.

Michels RG, Wilkinson CP, Rice TA: *Retinal Detachment.* St Louis: CV Mosby Co; 1990.

Norton EWD: Intraocular gas in the management of selected retinal detachments. XXIX Edward Jackson Memorial Lecture. *Trans Am Acad Ophthalmol Otolaryngol* 1973;77:OP85–98.

Norton EWD: Retinal detachment in aphakia. *Trans Am Ophthalmol Soc* 1963;61:770–789.

Norton EWD, Aaberg T, Fung W, et al: Giant retinal tears, I: clinical management with intravitreal air. *Am J Ophthalmol* 1969;68: 1011–1021.

Retina Society Terminology Committee. The classification of retinal detachment with proliferative vitreoretinopathy. *Ophthalmology* 1983;90:121–125.

Robertson DM: Delayed absorption of subretinal fluid after scleral buckling procedures. *Trans Am Ophthalmol Soc* 1978;76:557–583.

Ryan SJ, ed: *Retina*. Vol 3: *Surgical Retina*. St Louis: CV Mosby Co; 1989.

Schepens CL: *Retinal Detachment and Allied Diseases*. Philadelphia: WB Saunders Co; 1983: vols 1, 2.

Tornambe PE, Hilton GF, The Retinal Detachment Study Group: Pneumatic retinopexy: a multicenter randomized controlled clinical trial comparing pneumatic retinopexy and scleral buckling. *Ophthalmology* 1989;96:772–783.

Watzke RC: Scleral staphylomas and retinal detachment. *Arch Ophthalmol* 1963;70:796–804.

Zauberman H, Garcia RF: Treatment of retinal detachment without inducing chorioretinal lesions. *Trans Am Acad Ophthalmol Otolaryngol* 1975;79:OP835–844.

CHAPTER 7

Postoperative Management

The final anatomic result is rarely influenced by postoperative management, as most cases are cured in the operating room. However, the surgeon must be considerate of the patient's comfort and be alert for possible postoperative complications.

7-1

POSTOPERATIVE ORDERS

All surgeons cannot be expected to use the same postoperative orders, but the following (by G.F.H.) have been found to be satisfactory for patients who have undergone scleral buckling under general anesthesia. These orders assume postoperative hospitalization for 18 to 24 hours. Currently, however, many surgeons discharge selected patients several hours after surgery.

1. Clear liquid diet; progress to regular diet as tolerated
2. Bathroom privileges, with assistance as needed
3. May lie on unoperated side or on back
4. Meperidine (Demerol), 50 mg every 4 hours as needed for severe pain
5. Propoxyphene napsylate with acetaminophen (Darvocet-N 100), one every 4 hours as needed for moderate pain
6. Chloral hydrate, 500 mg at bedtime as needed; may repeat once
7. Prochlorperazine (Compazine), 10 mg every 4 hours as needed for nausea
8. Laxative of choice, once a day as needed
9. Bedside box with eight eyepads, paper tape 1 inch wide, 0.25% scopolamine, and Maxitrol solution
10. Ambulation: walk in hall first postoperative day

Nausea and vomiting are still unsolved problems for many patients who have had general anesthesia. Therefore, a clear liquid diet is indicated until the patient can tolerate the preoperative diet. An antiemetic, such as prochlorperazine, may be helpful.

Except in some cases of giant retinal breaks, total body rest is not required, and the patient may have bathroom privileges. Unless gas has been injected into the vitreous, it is usually not necessary for the patient to maintain a set head position, but it does seem that chemosis and lid edema are minimized if the patient rests on the unoperated side. It is generally acknowledged that ocular rest encourages the absorption of subretinal fluid. Most patients do well with patching of the affected eye only. If prolonged bed rest with critical positioning is required—for example, in certain cases with intravitreal gas—the possibility of thrombophlebitis is minimized by the use of elastic stockings and appropriate leg exercises.

Pain is rarely a problem for retinal patients. Meperidine, 50 to 100 mg, is seldom required beyond the first postoperative day. Propoxyphene napsylate with acetaminophen is an adequate analgesic thereafter.

As with many other inpatients, bowel function is often a preoccupation. A standing order for the laxative of choice saves the surgeon many phone calls, and routine orders might include "enema as needed."

Early ambulation has greatly minimized the postoperative problems of retinal patients. Decubitus ulcers, thrombophlebitis, and generalized weakness can be easily prevented by a program of ambulation commencing with a walk in the hall.

Antibiotics and corticosteroids, either topical or systemic, are not mandatory for routine cases, but many surgeons prefer a combination of drugs such as Maxitrol solution three times a day. Topical 0.25% scopolamine at the conclusion of surgery is usually sufficient to provide cycloplegia into the first postoperative day. The eye should be examined on the first postoperative day.

7-2

POSTOPERATIVE PHOTOCOAGULATION

Persistent leakage of fluid through a retinal break is usually an indication for reoperation, but occasionally the problem can be managed simply with postoperative photocoagulation. This treatment is not effective if the retinal break is significantly elevated from the retinal pigment epithelium; but if the break is only minimally elevated, photocoagulation should be considered. The goal of treatment is to induce swelling of the retina and choroid, thereby closing the edges of the break and allowing the subretinal fluid to be absorbed (Figure 7-1) and adhesions to permanently seal the break. When photocoagulation is to be performed, it is recommended that the physician patch the patient bilaterally and restrict activity before the procedure to encourage as much settling as possible. This may be done on an outpatient basis.

Even though argon laser photocoagulation is frequently applied with topical anesthesia only, retrobulbar anesthesia may be employed because of the tenderness of the postoperative eye. The surgeon may use either the slit lamp with a three-mirror

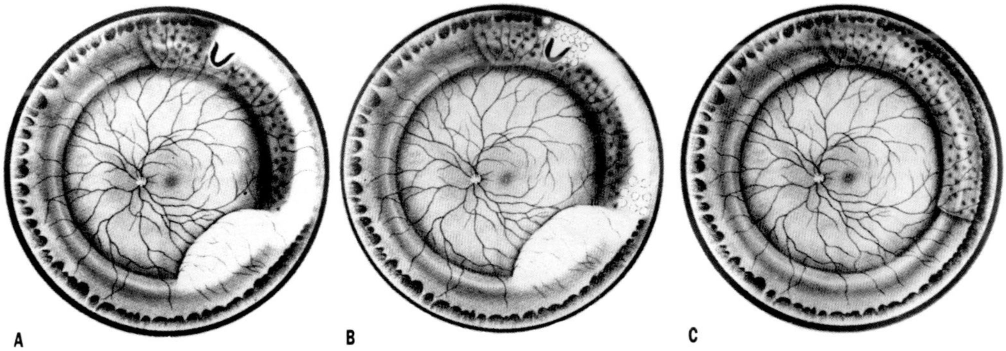

Figure 7-1 *Postoperative photocoagulation. (A) Inferior leakage of subretinal fluid, anteriorly from horseshoe break and across buckle in inferior temporal quadrant. (B) Photocoagulation around horseshoe tear and at 3:30-o'clock position. (C) Reattachment of retina after photocoagulation.*

contact lens or the laser indirect ophthalmoscope. Confluent treatment should be applied. The end point for treatment is prominent whitening of the retina. Two or three rows of contiguous lesions should be placed around the leaking break.

Maximal restriction of activity and proper positioning following supplemental laser application may preclude the need for surgical reoperation in some cases. If the response to treatment is not adequate, the surgeon should not hesitate to proceed with either pneumatic retinopexy or revision of the buckle.

7-3

POSTOPERATIVE PNEUMATIC RETINOPEXY

If there is too much subretinal fluid to be managed with photocoagulation, one may consider pneumatic retinopexy (see Section 6-2-3). Gas injection can be done on the ward or in the surgeon's office. If the break has remained open for more than 4 days after surgery, photocoagulation should be applied around the break after the retina has been pneumatically reattached.

7-4

DISCHARGE INSTRUCTIONS

The steady decrease in the duration of hospitalization during the last 20 years has not compromised the overall cure rate. Indeed, many scleral buckle operations are now performed in ambulatory surgery centers. At the time of discharge, it is useful to supply the patient with written postoperative instructions. Most of these limitations are arbitrary, but it is valuable to provide written instructions so that the surgeon, office staff, nursing personnel, and patient's family will all have reference to the same information. Expecting uniform agreement among surgeons regarding postoperative restrictions is not reasonable; however, those (by G.F.H.) listed below have been found to be satisfactory and are intended to be followed for 2 weeks.

1. Avoid stooping, bending, lifting anything weighing more than 10 pounds, and bumping your head.

2. Avoid sleeping on the side of the operated eye for 1 week.

3. You may shave after the second day.

4. You may watch television or read within the limits of comfort.

5. You may drink alcoholic beverages in moderation.

6. Avoid sexual intercourse.

7. You may bathe the eyelids daily with cotton or gauze moistened with warm tap water. Do not bathe the eyeball itself.

8. Some discharge from the operated eye is to be expected. This should show gradual improvement. If you develop any difficulty during the postoperative period, contact the physician's office.

9. Change the eyepad at least daily. Clear plastic tape or paper tape may be used to hold the pad in position. You may discontinue use of the eyepad whenever it is comfortable to do so (approximately 6 days after surgery).

10. Medication instructions:

- Scopolamine 0.25% (red-topped plastic container): one drop in the operated eye at bedtime.
- Maxitrol (white-topped container): one drop in the operated eye three times a day.
- Propoxyphene napsylate with acetaminophen (Darvocet-N 100): one tablet every 4 hours as needed for pain; if not adequate, call the office.
- Other: ______________________

11. Return appointment: ______________

The majority of patients probably would have a satisfactory surgical result without most of the restrictions. However, imposing them routinely seems justified because they can be important for the occasional patient. In addition, moderate limitations appear to enhance the psychological security of the patient.

The presence of subretinal fluid should not postpone discharge from the hospital. There may be persistent fluid inferiorly for several weeks.

Generally, the restrictions may be discontinued 2 weeks after the operation. The majority of patients are able to return to work within 2 or 3 weeks; but if a patient's occupation requires clear binocular vision, convalescence is longer. Further restrictions are not indicated, but young patients should be counseled to avoid contact sports, such as boxing or tackle football.

7-5

FOLLOWUP EXAMINATIONS

The routine patient should be examined on the first day after surgery, at 1, 3, and 6 weeks, and at 3, 6, and 12 months, after which annual examinations are recommended. More frequent examinations are necessary if complications develop. Examination should include an interval history, best corrected visual acuity, tonometry, biomicroscopy, and thorough binocular indirect ophthalmoscopy. Routine examination of the contralateral fundus should not be neglected.

If eyeglasses were worn preoperatively, they will suffice for visual acuity measurements, with a pinhole as indicated, in the early postoperative period. The refractive error generally stabilizes in 3 months and, if indicated, a permanent spectacle lens may be ordered at that time. Maximum recovery of visual acuity generally occurs within 6 months, but occasionally a patient notes some improvement in acuity for 1 to 2 years. Retinal reattachment surgery often has a marked effect on scleral rigidity. Therefore, instead of indentation tonometry, applanation tonometry is recommended. The anterior chamber reaction revealed by biomicroscopy is usually mild, and daily use of a cycloplegic and an antibiotic-corticosteroid combination for 2 weeks is sufficient. In the occasional case in which significant inflammation is noted, appropriate corticosteroid medication should prescribed. Scleral indentation is not generally recommended for the first 2 weeks after surgery. Annual examinations help assure the discovery of such asymptomatic problems as new retinal breaks, peripheral detachment, erosion of the implant, or glaucoma.

SUGGESTED READINGS

Burton TC, Arafat NL, Phelps CD: Intraocular pressure in retinal detachment. *Int Ophthalmol* 1979;1:147–152.

McMeel JW, Wapner JM: Infections and retinal surgery. *Arch Ophthalmol* 1965;74:42–47.

Michels RG: Scleral buckling methods for rhegmatogenous retinal detachment. *Retina* 1986;6:1–49.

Pemberton JW: Schiotz-applanation disparity following retinal detachment surgery. *Arch Ophthalmol* 1969;81:534–537.

Phelps CD, Burton TC: Glaucoma and retinal detachment. *Arch Ophthalmol* 1977;95:418–422.

CHAPTER 8

Complications of Reattachment Surgery

Serious complications of retinal detachment surgery are infrequent, occurring in less than 10% of cases. The discussion of complications in this chapter is limited to those of the scleral buckling operation and occurrences that have potentially adverse effects on the performance of the surgery, the prognosis for reattachment, the health of the eye, or anticipated effects on eye function. (For references to the literature on complications of the alternative procedures discussed in Section 6-2, see the Suggested Readings at the end of Chapters 6 and 8.)

8-1

INTRAOPERATIVE COMPLICATIONS

Complications that sometimes develop during surgery include corneal epithelial edema, miosis, bleeding into the anterior chamber, perforation or rupture of the sclera, intraocular hemorrhage, choroidal detachment, incarceration of the retina, retinal break, vitreous loss, elevated intraocular pressure, and the complications of an intraocular injection, such as cataract, retinal perforation, or vitreous hemorrhage.

8-1-1 Corneal Complications

Corneal epithelial edema or trauma to the epithelium impairs the clarity of the cornea and impedes optimal visualization of the retina at surgery. Several factors are responsible for a majority of the cases. It is routine in some operating rooms to instill preoperative topical anesthetics for eye surgery. This practice should not be allowed for retinal detachment surgery, because topical anesthetics adversely affect the epithelium.

For the same reason, concentrated detergents should not be used in the surgical preparation. Prolonged exposure to detergents leads to desiccation of the epithelium, and undue global pressure at surgery results in edema of the epithelium, especially in elderly adults with an aging endothelium and in diabetic patients. Most cases respond well to mechanical expression of the edema fluid. This is accomplished by firmly pressing on the limbus with a dry, cotton-tipped applicator. The applicator is then rolled across the cornea. This maneuver expresses the edema but does not remove the epithelium. In persistent cases of epithelial edema, the central portion of the epithelium must be removed with gentle strokes of a tilted knife blade, avoiding damage to Bowman's membrane.

8-1-2 Pupillary Complications

Infrequently, there is minimal bleeding into the anterior chamber. As the blood settles onto the anterior lens capsule, the view of the fundus is obscured. A clear view can be regained by pushing the blood into the chamber angle by means of an intracameral injection of sodium hyaluronate (Healon).

Intraoperative miosis is due most commonly to hypotony. Intravitreal gas that comes in contact with the iris can also cause miosis. If the pupil does not dilate with cycloplegic and mydriatic drops, intracameral epinephrine may be considered.

8-1-3 Scleral Complications

Rarely, inadvertent perforation of the sclera occurs during surgery due either to excessively deep placement of a suture needle or to excessively deep lamellar dissection in preparing the implant site. In either case, the retina must be inspected immediately to determine if associated iatrogenic perforation of the retina has occurred. If it has, the retinal perforation site must be treated with cryotherapy or diathermy, and the scleral buckle must be shifted or modified as needed to position the new break optimally on the buckle. If the perforation occurred in an area of attached retina, vitreous may be present in the perforation site, whereas perforation in the area of the detachment prematurely releases subretinal fluid. Hypotony results, making further suturing difficult and increasing the risk of a second perforation or a choroidal hemorrhage. Less frequently, inadvertent scleral perforation occurs during a maneuver close to or involving the sclera—for example, in tenotomy of an extraocular muscle, sharp dissection to lyse episcleral adhesions, or revision of previous intrascleral implant sites.

Perhaps the most disastrous, but fortunately rare, complication is forceful rupture of the sclera. The combination of excessive traction by the traction sutures, increased intraocular pressure, and thin sclera (as in staphyloma, the bed of a previous implant, or thin bed of a new implant) results in rupture of the sclera at its weakest point, with abrupt herniation of choroid, retina, and, frequently, vitreous. Ophthalmoscopic examination of the retina is imperative. Repair of the rupture requires closure of the scleral flaps, a scleral patch over the area, or scleral imbrication. Cryosurgical treatment should be applied cautiously, and the scleral buckle should be positioned to overlie the rupture site. The prognosis for successful reattachment is significantly worse following rupture of the sclera.

8-1-4 Choroidal Complications

Hemorrhage is the major complication involving the choroid. During drainage of subretinal fluid, hemorrhage at the perforation can result in free bleeding into the subretinal or suprachoroidal spaces. In a case in which the macula is detached, the blood may pool in the posterior pole beneath the macula. If the blood has not yet reached the macula, proper postoperative positioning of the patient to allow the blood to gravitate away from the macula can minimize permanent adverse effects on visual acuity. The surgery is further complicated if the hemorrhage gains access to the vitreous via the retinal breaks, markedly reducing visibility. Occasionally, the choroidal hemorrhage remains confined to the choroid or the suprachoroidal space. This does not usually hinder the surgery unless the hemorrhage becomes massive or interferes with subsequent placement of treatment. Hemorrhages of this type may ensue premature removal of the cryoprobe while it is still frozen to the sclera and choroid. Manipulation of the probe fractures the frozen choroid, which hemorrhages when it thaws. Choroidal hemorrhaging is more common in high myopia. Serous choroidal detachment may be differentiated from hemorrhagic choroidal detachment with intraoperative transillumination of the globe.

8-1-5 Retinal Complications

During surgery, the retina per se is not directly manipulated; it is only secondarily influenced by the maneuvers of the procedure. Consequently, retinal complications are uncommon. The retina may become incarcerated during inadvertent scleral perforation or scleral rupture. More common is incarceration of the retina into the drainage site on release of subretinal fluid. Excessive pressure on the globe during perforation for drainage allows egress of subretinal fluid to occur too rapidly, which may cause the retina to be drawn to the perforation site and incarcerated. Premature and sudden cessation of subretinal fluid flow during drainage should alert the surgeon to this possibility. It should be confirmed by re-examination of the retina for radiating retinal folds drawn to the site of perforation. Repeated perforation at the same site should never be attempted. Gentle external massage over the perforation site to free the retina internally is a tempting but futile maneuver, because it does not release the retina. The prognosis is not adversely affected unless a retinal fold extends to the macula or to an adjacent retinal break. Incarceration may be accompanied by a new retinal break due to rupture. New breaks may also result from perforation of the retina with the drainage needle or scleral suture needle.

8-1-6 Vitreal Complications

Egress of a small bead of vitreous at surgery is a serious complication. If the egress is massive, as it can be when the sclera ruptures, additional complications may develop. The problem is not the lost vitreous per se but the secondary alterations in the remaining vitreous. As vitreous gel shifts toward the perforation or rupture site, vitreoretinal adhesions are stressed throughout the retina, and vitreous may be present in the subretinal space. Both conditions prevent satisfactory settling of the detached retina on the scleral buckle, and it may be impossible to adequately reapproximate open breaks on the buckle to obtain a subsequent cure. Vitrectomy may be required at reoperation.

A further complication during surgery is loss of media transparency due to hemorrhage into the vitreous. Even a small hemorrhage dispersed into the vitreous from the site of subretinal fluid drainage appreciably reduces the visibility of retinal details. Fortunately, this complication develops late in the procedure, after treatment has been applied and the scleral buckle positioned. Despite the loss of visibility, the operation can usually be successfully completed and the hemorrhage clears postoperatively.

8-1-7 Elevated Intraocular Pressure

Most retinal detachment procedures have some effect on the intraocular pressure. Pressure on the globe with the cryoprobe or drainage of subretinal fluid leads to hypotony, while scleral buckling, diathermy, and intraocular injections contribute to increased intraocular pressure. It is usually possible to adjust the intraocular pressure to near-normal levels by the time surgery is completed if subretinal fluid has been drained. In nondrainage scleral buckling procedures, the pressure is temporarily elevated but will not present a problem if the central retinal artery is open and carefully monitored. Excessive increase in intraocular pressure leads to closure of the central retinal artery. Therefore, prolonged and excessive traction on the traction sutures or compression of the globe should be avoided. The retinal arterial circulation must be examined frequently to make sure that the central retinal artery has not been closed by increased intraocular pressure during adjustment of scleral buckle tension, while tightening of sutures, or after an intraocular injection.

8-1-8 Complications of Intraocular Injections

In cases requiring drainage of large amounts of subretinal fluid, it may be necessary to restore the intraocular volume with sterile air, gas, or balanced salt solution. The injection procedure is not without hazard and should not be used indiscriminately or routinely. The first complication encountered is tenting of the pars plana epithelium by the tip of the advancing needle, with the subsequent passage of the injection into the subretinal space instead of the vitreous cavity. This complication can be avoided by ophthalmoscopic observation of the needle tip before injection to ascertain that the tip has, in fact, perforated the pars plana epithelium and vitreous base as intended. Stable fixation of the globe during the procedure is mandatory to prevent inadvertent rotation of the globe that brings the lens or retina in contact with the needle. Minimal contact of the needle with the lens may result in corresponding linear opacities in the posterior capsule, which may be transient. More forceful contact produces permanent opacification of the lens.

The injection per se may lead to additional complications. Injected intraocular solutions, being incompressible fluids within a confined space, create a high pressure rise toward the end of maximum injection. Excess injection of as little as 0.2 ml is sufficient to raise the intraocular pressure well above the perfusion pressure of the central retinal artery, with resultant closure of the artery. In contrast to injected solutions, sterile air is compressible and causes Schiotz tonometry to be falsely low. Improper air injection technique can result in myriad minute bubbles ("fish eggs"), which temporarily obscure further visualization of retinal details. Aside from immediate complications of intraocular injections, the possible later development of endophthalmitis must be kept in mind. (For a discussion of endophthalmitis, see Section 8-2-2-5.)

8-2

EARLY POSTOPERATIVE COMPLICATIONS

Complications that arise during the first 10 days after surgery can be classified as early postoperative. During this period, a certain amount of pain, lid edema, chemosis, orbital edema, and haziness of the intraocular media is accepted as normal. Most early complications begin with accentuation of one of these conditions, and differentiation between the expected course and complications can be difficult. If development of a complication is suspected, it is essential to determine and document the trend of the course by specific examination several times during the next 12 to 24 hours. Corrective therapy must be instituted early. Whereas the course of the few normal postoperative conditions is generally toward spontaneous resolution, complications become progressively worse.

8-2-1 Systemic Complications

The range of possible systemic complications occurring postoperatively is extensive, but their incidence is fortunately uncommon. Some are related to the stress of anesthesia and surgery, others to age and the patient's physical status before surgery. In elderly patients, mental disorientation can pose a serious hazard and requires nearly constant nursing attention.

Adequate hydration, omission or reduction of sedatives and narcotics, avoidance of bilateral patches, and contact with family help restore mentation. If the operated eye is the patient's only useful eye, postoperative patching should be minimal to allow visual sensory input to help reestablish orientation.

Early postoperative ambulation has significantly reduced the occurrence of pulmonary embolism, but the complication remains a possibility in predisposed patients. Current management of retinal detachment seldom necessitates immobilization and prolonged bed rest, which can lead to pulmonary embolism.

Rarely, elderly patients suffer myocardial infarction in the early postoperative period. Specific preoperative evaluation of cardiac status and the risk to the patient is prudent. The decision for surgery must be carefully weighed in high-risk cardiac patients. A seemingly healthy patient can develop a myocardial infarction and arrest within a few days after surgery, requiring emergency treatment and appropriate management by a medical consultant.

Acute postoperative urinary retention secondary to benign prostatic hypertrophy is not uncommon following general anesthesia. Fortunately, palliative treatment with a catheter is effective and does not interfere with the ocular management, but prostatectomy may be required at a later time. Of more serious consequence is the very rare postoperative complication of acute renal failure occurring in predisposed patients—for example, individuals with diabetes. Again, the preoperative medical evaluation should detect high-risk patients with renal compromise, and the findings should be considered in the recommendation regarding surgery.

8-2-2 Ocular Complications

Early postoperative ocular complications include conjunctival adhesions, anterior segment ischemia, increased intraocular pressure, vitreous opacification, endophthalmitis, choroidal detachment, and exudative redetachment.

8-2-2-1 Conjunctival Adhesions After retinal detachment surgery, conjunctival adhesions occasionally develop. Adhesion formation appears to be related to the extent of surgery, the amount of reactive orbital swelling, and the inadvertent freezing of conjunctiva during surgery. An adhesion between bulbar and palpebral conjunctiva will become a permanent symblepharon if not treated early. Each day the recurring adhesion must be lysed with a smooth glass rod or a muscle-hook tip. In the absence of a glass rod, a simple fever thermometer may be used. Topical anesthesia, such as 4% lidocaine, should be administered. Applications of ointment into the cul-de-sac help prevent other adhesions.

8-2-2-2 Anterior Segment Ischemia Ischemia of the anterior segment is a consequence of impaired blood flow in the long posterior ciliary arteries and anterior ciliary arteries to the ciliary body and iris. A massive exudation occurs in the anterior segment, with associated inflammatory response.

Clinically, the syndrome is recognized by pain, corneal edema, folds in Descemet's membrane, proteinaceous flare, cells in the anterior chamber, keratic precipitates, edema of the iris, transillumination defects of the iris pigment epithelium, cataract, and increased or decreased intraocular pressure.

The ischemia results from the surgical technique of retinal reattachment and is most closely related to the number of rectus muscles removed, the inadvertent treatment of long posterior ciliary arteries with diathermy, or the tight, narrow encircling elements. Each contributes to obstructive compromise of circulation to the anterior uvea. Infrequently, tenotomy of one rectus muscle is required to facilitate access; rarely, two may be removed—but never three. To avoid the long posterior ciliary arteries, diathermy treatment should not be placed in the 3- and 9-o'clock meridians. Highly elevated, narrow scleral buckles are inadvisable. As a result of increased awareness of these caveats, the complication has become very rare.

An additional factor precipitating or aggravating anterior segment ischemia is the presence of blood dyscrasias or hemoglobinopathies with intravascular clotting phenomena. The prime example is SC sickle cell hemoglobinopathy. SC patients should have an exchange blood transfusion preoperatively to increase the normal A-hemoglobin, as determined by electrophoresis, to at least 60%. Local anesthesia is preferred, and oxygen should be given throughout the procedure. Postoperatively, SC patients may benefit from supplemental oxygen for 24 to 48 hours.

Corrective treatment of ischemia should be started early. However, the results of treatment are often disappointing. Systemic and topical corticosteroids, cycloplegic medications, and removal of a tight scleral buckle constitute the treatment.

8-2-2-3 Increased Intraocular Pressure During the early postoperative period, the detection of corneal epithelial edema, pain, or pulsation of the central retinal artery is usually grounds for suspecting increased intraocular pressure. Patients likely to develop the complication include narrow-angle glaucoma suspects, elderly patients with enlarged lenses, those who have subluxated lenses, patients with pre-existing open-angle glaucoma, those who received relatively large injections of intraocular gas, and especially those with prominent postoperative choroidal detachment that has produced shallowing of the anterior chamber with closure of the angle. Moderate elevations to 30 mm Hg are frequently transient and usually do not require treatment. Higher pressures may be due to some degree of angle closure. The condition is usually self-limiting and responds well to acetazolamide (Diamox). The most common causative mechanism is anterior displacement of the lens and iris by the presence of choroidal detachment and subsequent compromise of the filtration angle. Topical corticosteroids can discourage the development of peripheral anterior synechiae. If the administration of acetazolamide, timolol, epinephrine, hyperosmotic agents, systemic corticosteroids, or cycloplegic drops fails to control the pressure, and the filtration angle is obscured by peripheral iris, it may be necessary to drain the choroidal detachment via posterior sclerotomies to reopen the angle and prevent permanent anterior synechiae.

8-2-2-4 Vitreous Opacification Although the majority of cases retain relatively clear vitreous postoperatively, a few develop rapidly progressive opacification of the vitreous. The cause is unknown, but extensively treated cases are likely to have sustained significant tissue injury, which excites a sterile inflammatory response with cells and proteinaceous exudation into the vitreous. Although the opacification may become dense, it responds to a short-term course of systemic corticosteroids and in most cases leaves little residual opacity. Occasionally, as a consequence of the intense inflammatory process, transvitreal membranes and strands develop and subsequently lead to sufficient traction to redetach the retina. If the traction responsible for the redetachment is limited, reoperation with revision of the buckle will suffice; but if the traction is extensive, vitrectomy should be considered.

8-2-2-5 Endophthalmitis Bacterial endophthalmitis is a rare complication following retinal detachment surgery and implies a direct inoculum of sufficient bacteria to propagate. Possible routes of infection include the perforation site for draining subretinal fluid, accidental rupture of the globe, the injection of intraocular air, gas, or balanced salt solution, and areas of exposed choroid in the bed of an intrascleral buckle. Lengthy procedures, extensive scleral surgery, reoperation, and multiple drainage attempts also increase the risk of bacterial contamination and postoperative endophthalmitis.

The earliest clinical symptoms and signs, developing by the third to fifth postoperative day, are pain, chemosis, lid edema, the appearance of localized vitreous opacification or petechial hemorrhages, and acute subretinal exudates at the level of the scleral buckle, noticeable in an examination by indirect ophthalmoscopy. The recognition of such symptoms and signs is critical to proper management of endophthalmitis, for retinal damage is rapid, and soon the vitreous becomes opaque with inflammatory reaction. Systemic corticosteroids without antibiotics may be mistakenly initiated, on the incorrect assumption that the process is sterile.

If intraocular infection with vitreous involvement may be present, vitreous cultures must be obtained immediately, followed by intravitreal antibiotic injection. Intravitreal corticosteroid injection is controversial. The indications for vitrectomy also remain controversial, but immediate vitrectomy should probably be performed if vitreous involvement is moderate or severe. If the scleral buckle is implicated, it must be removed, along with all sutures. Subconjunctival antibiotics are injected and broad-spectrum systemic antibiotics are started immediately, as well as topical fortified antibiotics, cycloplegics, and corticosteroids. Specific antibiotics can be selected after culture identification of the organism and determination of the sensitivity to antibiotics. Depending on clinical response, subsequent vitreous cultures and intravitreal antibiotic injection should be considered within 48 hours.

The prognosis for successful reattachment of the retina and a satisfactory functional result in the presence of bacterial endophthalmitis is generally very poor, but it depends on the virulence of the organism. If the infection is entirely extraocular, involving the buckle but without any sign of endophthalmitis, intravitreal injections are not indicated. The buckle should be removed, along with all sutures, and systemic, subconjunctival, and topical antibiotics should be administered.

8-2-2-6 Choroidal Detachment In approximately 5% to 10% of scleral buckling procedures, some degree of choroidal detachment develops secondary to fluid accumulation in the suprachoroidal space. The fluid is assumed to be a transudation from the choroid. Its formation is related in part to advanced age and in part to surgical factors, such as thermal treatment, trauma to the choroid, hypotony, and obstruction of vortex vein outflow (particularly with very broad buckles) with resultant increased intravascular pressure throughout the choroidal vascular system. Although care is taken at surgery to minimize the procedural factors, choroidal detachment is still a postoperative problem. In a majority of cases, the overlying retina remains in satisfactory apposition to the treated retinal pigment epithelium, and because of eventual spontaneous resolution of the choroidal detachment, the prognosis is usually good.

A more serious complication is choroidal detachment into large bullae with closure of the filtration angle as the ciliary body is rotated anteriorly at the scleral spur. The situation can usually be managed medically, but occasionally corrective surgical intervention is necessary to prevent permanent synechial closure of the filtration angle and glaucoma. Topical corticosteroids may minimize synechia formation, but no medication is entirely effective in influencing the choroidal detachment. At reoperation, it is necessary to drain the suprachoroidal fluid via sclerotomies and restore the intraocular volume by injecting balanced salt solution. Despite some reaccumulation of fluid, the operation is usually successful.

Massive detachments of the choroid may actually touch in the central vitreous ("kissing choroidals"). The problem requires surgical drainage to prevent the possibility of adhesion of retina to retina with subsequent tractional retinal redetachment.

Hemorrhagic choroidal detachments are less frequent than the common serous detachment, and the prognosis is poorer. The loculated hemorrhage is analogous to a hematoma elsewhere. The majority of cases follow a self-limiting course to spontaneous resolution, but some have considerable chronic inflammatory response characterized by proteinaceous transudation, opacification of the vitreous, glaucoma, and occasional failure of the retina to reattach successfully. In some cases, the hemorrhage passes through the retina to produce a dense vitreous hemorrhage.

8-2-2-7 Exudative Redetachment Rarely, thermal treatment of the choroid leads to postoperative transudation into the subretinal space and extensive secondary redetachment of the retina 2 to 3 days after surgery. Providing the retinal breaks remain in apposition to the scleral buckle, the secondary detachment resolves in 2 to 12 weeks in a majority of cases. The secondary subretinal fluid does not usually communicate with the retinal breaks and remains posterior to the scleral buckle, which accounts for the good prognosis. These postoperative detachments frequently are signified by "shifting fluid."

8-3

LATE POSTOPERATIVE COMPLICATIONS

Complications classified as late postoperative are those that occur more than 10 days after surgery.

8-3-1 Persistent Ocular Pain

Besides the expected postoperative discomfort of surgery, some patients experience persistent ocular or cephalic pain for weeks or months after surgery. The effects of surgery have healed, the retina has been reattached, and the eye is without inflammation, yet the pain persists. The cause has not been determined, but the pain may be due to persistent irritation by the scleral buckle of adjacent afferent branches of the long posterior ciliary nerve in its intrascleral course. Long-term analgesic medication is not entirely effective or feasible. Retrobulbar lidocaine, repeated several times, may interrupt the pain pattern and produce permanent relief. A retrobulbar injection of 50% alcohol and 50% lidocaine provides relief from pain for as long as several months. Despite a satisfactory anatomic and functional result, persistent pain may eventually dictate removal of the scleral buckle.

8-3-2 Infection

The various implant materials and sutures used in retinal detachment surgery are foreign bodies and can become nidi for infection. The organisms responsible are frequently coagulase-positive staphylococci but may be Gram-negative bacteria. The incidence varies, depending on the surgical technique and observance of the principles of asepsis. The major clinical indication is pain, which should be considered a symptom of infection until proved otherwise. Other signs to look for are inflammation of the conjunctiva, subconjunctival hemorrhage, point tenderness, purulent discharge, and occasionally a draining of the sinus tract through the conjunctiva. Fortunately, associated intraocular involvement is rare, but its existence must be definitely ruled out. Normally, the scleral buckling material becomes enveloped within a connective tissue sheath, which develops soon after the initial buckling procedure. Therefore, a potential space exists for invasion of organisms between the buckle material and the tissue sheath over the entire extent of the buckle.

For infections diagnosed after the first postoperative month, treatment consists of removal of the scleral buckle, identification of the organism, and appropriate antibiotics. For extraocular infections occurring within the first postoperative month, medical treatment may be administered to suppress the infection and gain sufficient time for the retina to firmly reattach before the scleral buckle is removed. Any evidence of intraocular extension of infection, however, demands immediate removal of the buckle. When the retina has been completely reattached, removal of the buckle only infrequently leads to redetachment. A second scleral buckling procedure, if required for detachment, may be undertaken as soon as all evidence of residual infection has disappeared.

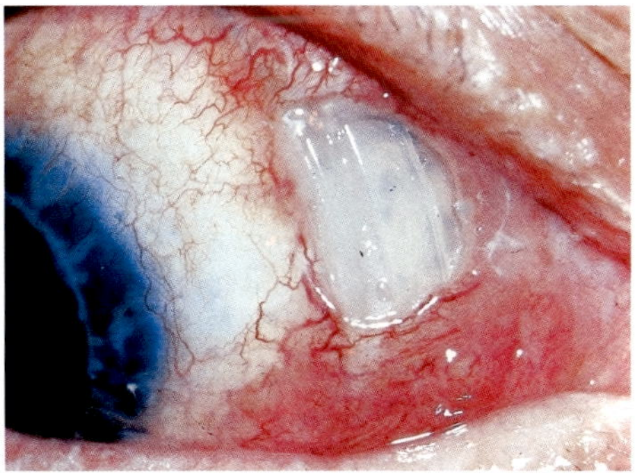

Figure 8-1 *Erosion of silicone through Tenon's capsule and conjunctiva.*
Courtesy Lawrence Lonn, MD.

8-3-3 Exposure of Scleral Buckle

As a consequence of infection or inadequate coverage of scleral implants at surgery, segments of buckle material may erode through overlying Tenon's capsule and conjunctiva (Figure 8-1). Clinical signs of bacterial infection may or may not be present. Providing the retina is well attached, there is no advantage in attempting to modify the scleral buckle or to patch over the exposed portion. Encircling elements and well-covered intrascleral implants rarely become exposed, because they have no free ends that can come loose and have the inherent advantage of conforming to the globe. But segmental episcleral buckles have a greater tendency to erode through overlying Tenon's capsule and conjunctiva. Most exposed buckles eventually have to be removed. Indications for removal include clinical infection, pain, or a cosmetic problem.

8-3-4 Migration or Intrusion of Scleral Buckle

At the time of surgery, care should be taken to place adequate anchoring sutures in each quadrant. Otherwise, the encircling band, being under tension, has a natural tendency to slip anteriorly or posteriorly. With anterior migration, the band has, in rare cases, eroded through the insertions of the rectus muscles, with subsequent erosion through conjunctiva. Posterior migration may progressively compromise the macula and optic nerve.

A related complication is intrusion of the encircling element into the globe. The mechanism is purely mechanical. The narrow band, under circumferential tension, gradually erodes through sclera, choroid, pigment epithelium, and retina, eventually to lie in the vitreous. This complication was most commonly seen with encircling polyethylene tubes or the Arruga string circlage used in the past; it has not been a frequent problem with current encircling materials. Progressive intrusion is insidious and may be advanced before the patient becomes aware of the complication. Hemorrhage into the vitreous or redetachment of the retina becomes apparent to the patient and precipitates discovery of the intrusion.

Surgical removal of the intruding buckle should be attempted only for recurrent retinal detachment or recurrent vitreous hemorrhage. Otherwise, the intrusion should be managed conservatively. Frequently, the band can remain in the subretinal space without causing further problems. Removal is hazardous to the eye, and the prognosis is unpredictable. In removing the intraocular portion of the intruded scleral buckle, the surgeon must identify the sites of buckle entry and exit at the sclera. The buckle should be cut cleanly at one site, and the element carefully extracted through the opposite site. No discontinuities such as abutted ends, sutures, or metal clips may be present along the intraocular portion, because they will tear the retina when attempts are made to extract the buckle. Scrupulous observance of aseptic technique is mandatory in these cases, because organisms can readily gain intraocular access. Alternatively, simple cutting of the encircling element may relieve the circumferential traction and eliminate the hazard of total removal.

8-3-5 Proliferative Vitreoretinopathy

The term *proliferative vitreoretinopathy* (PVR) connotes the pathologic process in which the formation of a membrane on the retinal and vitreal surfaces leads to contracture and precipitates redetachment of the retina. (For further discussion of PVR, see Section 2-9-3 and Section 3-16.) The process develops postoperatively in about 5% of retinal reattachment cases and accounts for almost all failed operations. Pre-existing uveitis, ocular trauma, hemorrhage, and intraoperative complications have been identified as contributing factors in the development of PVR and redetachment of the retina. PVR is usually extensive, is intimately associated with the retina, and carries a poor prognosis for reoperation. The clinical appearance of a fully developed case is that of a total retinal detachment with white, immobile, fixed folds of retina. Occasionally, PVR is localized to one quadrant or less. Pars plana vitrectomy, with removal or segmentation of the periretinal membranes and intraocular injection of gas or silicone oil, may be used in an attempt to resolve this complication.

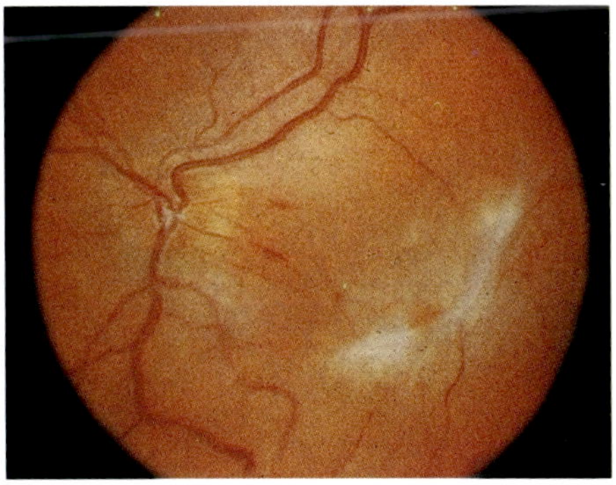

Figure 8-2 *Postoperative macular pucker.*

8-3-6 Macular Pucker

A preretinal membrane may pucker the macula and compromise vision (Figure 8-2). The presence of hemorrhage in the vitreous or vitreal membranes increases the chance of postoperative macular pucker. Macular preretinal membranes relax spontaneously in less than 1% of cases. Vision usually improves after vitrectomy and preretinal membrane removal in selected cases.

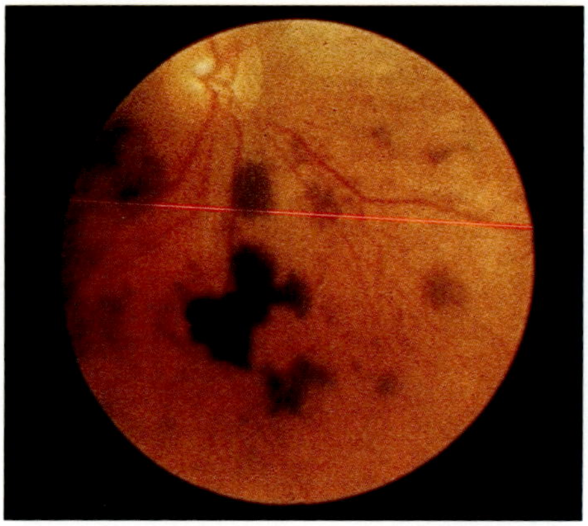

Figure 8-3 *Subretinal pigment migration ("fall-out") after cryosurgical retinal reattachment.*

8-3-7 Other Late Complications

Additional complications include secondary ptosis, enophthalmos, refractive changes, extraocular muscle imbalance, and optic atrophy. Ptosis of varying degrees may be associated with operative trauma to the levator muscle or its nerve, or it may represent pseudoptosis secondary to enophthalmos. Enophthalmos results from atrophy of orbital adipose tissue, allowing the globe to recede deeper within the orbit. Aside from cosmetic considerations, these findings do not adversely affect the functional result. A relative myopic refractive change is anticipated, especially in encircling procedures, but astigmatism may also occur. The induced anisometropia, with associated aniseikonia, may be symptomatic. During surgery, the extraocular muscles are subject to considerable mechanical trauma, which may compromise their actions postoperatively. Adhesion of muscles to the sclera posteriorly, accounting for limitation of full rotations, is uncommon after scleral buckling procedures, as is diplopia in the primary position. Strabismus surgery to lyse adhesions or alter muscle action is rarely necessary.

Cryotherapy applications may physically disrupt retinal pigment epithelial cells, thus releasing pigment into the subretinal fluid—referred to as "pigment fallout" (Figure 8-3). The amount of pigment released is directly related to the number and intensity of cryotherapy applications. When the macula is detached, there is a natural gravitational settling of the pigment near or at the fovea. A prospective study has demonstrated that the resultant visual acuity in such cases is no worse than in control cases and has concluded that the presence of subfoveal pigment does not impair visual function. This finding is in contrast to the detrimental effect of submacular hemorrhage on visual acuity.

8-4

INCIDENCE OF SCLERAL BUCKLING COMPLICATIONS

The complications listed in Table 8-1 were noted in a series of 1000 consecutive detachments operated on by one of the authors (G.F.H.). Some part of most of the operations was performed by a resident or fellow. Several complications occasionally occurred in a single eye.

The figure of 4.4% operative retinal breaks is high and probably reflects the fact that the data were generated in a teaching hospital. Fortunately, iatrogenic breaks are not serious, because they are nontractional, small holes and are readily closed. All 44 eyes with iatrogenic retinal breaks were reattached.

Of 26 eyes with retinal incarceration, 17 were reattached. The failures were due to PVR. A possible association between incarceration and PVR is unclear.

The effects of the hemorrhages were all transient except in 7 eyes: 4 had subretinal hemorrhage into the fovea; in 2, vitreous hemorrhages failed to clear (prior to the availability of vitrectomy); and in 1 case, hemorrhagic choroidal detachment resulted in permanent but controllable glaucoma.

Most problems of extraocular muscle imbalance were transient, but 4 patients required corrective muscle surgery.

TABLE 8-1

Complications of Scleral Buckling (1000 Eyes)

Complications	Percentage
Intraoperative	
Retinal break	4.4
Retinal incarceration	2.6
Retinal, choroidal, or vitreal hemorrhage	4.3
Vitreous loss	0.6
Rupture of globe	0.4
Choroidal detachment	0.9
Avulsion of extraocular muscle	0.2
Postoperative	
Choroidal detachment	6.1
Intraocular infection (presumed)	0.1
Extraocular infection	0.8
Exoplant exposure without infection	0.2
Severe uveitis	1.3
Increased intraocular pressure	1.3
Corneal problems	0.7
Proliferative vitreoretinopathy (PVR)	5.6
Macular pucker	1.6
Diplopia	3.6

SUGGESTED READINGS

Avins LR, Hilton GF: Lesions simulating serous detachment of the pigment epithelium: occurrence after retinal detachment surgery. *Arch Ophthalmol* 1980;98:1427–1429.

Burton TC, Arafat NL, Phelps CD: Intraocular pressure in retinal detachment. *Int Ophthalmol* 1979;1:147–152.

Flindall RJ, Norton EWD, Curtin VT, et al: Reduction of extrusion and infection following episcleral silicone implants and cryopexy in retinal detachment surgery. *Am J Ophthalmol* 1971;71:835–837.

Folk JC, Cutkomp J, Koontz FP: Bacterial abscesses after retinal buckling operations: pathogenesis, management, and laboratory investigations. *Ophthalmology* 1987;94:1148.

Hawkins WR, Schepens CL: Choroidal detachment and retinal surgery. *Am J Ophthalmol* 1966;62:813–819.

Hilton GF: Subretinal pigment migration following cryosurgical retinal reattachment. *Mod Probl Ophthalmol* 1974;12:64–70.

Hilton, GF, Grizzard WS, Avins LR, et al: The drainage of subretinal fluid: a randomized controlled clinical trial. *Retina* 1981;1:271–280.

Hilton GF, Tornambe PE, The Retinal Detachment Study Group: Pneumatic retinopexy: an analysis of intraoperative and postoperative complications [including anatomic results in 1274 eyes]. *Retina* 1991;11:285–294.

Hilton GF, Wallyn RH: The removal of scleral buckles. *Arch Ophthalmol* 1978;96:2061–2063.

Jarrett WH, Brockhurst RJ: Unexplained blindness and optic atrophy following retinal detachment surgery. *Arch Ophthalmol* 1965;73: 782–791.

Lobes LA Jr, Burton TC: The incidence of macular pucker after retinal detachment surgery. *Am J Ophthalmol* 1978;85:72–77.

Lobes LA Jr, Grand MG: Incidence of cystoid macular edema following scleral buckling procedure. *Arch Ophthalmol* 1980;98:1230–1232.

McMeel JW, Wapner JM: Infections and retinal surgery. *Arch Ophthalmol* 1965;74:42–47.

Packer AJ, Maggiano JM, Aaberg TM, et al: Serous choroidal detachment after retinal detachment surgery. *Arch Ophthalmol* 1983; 101:1221–1224.

Pemberton JW: Schiotz-applanation disparity following retinal detachment surgery. *Arch Ophthalmol* 1969;81:534–537.

Phelps CD, Burton TC: Glaucoma and retinal detachment. *Arch Ophthalmol* 1977;95:418–422.

Regan CDJ, Schepens CL: Erosion of the ocular wall by circling polyethylene tubing: a late complication of scleral buckling. *Am J Ophthalmol* 1964;57:79–83.

Robertson DM: Delayed absorption of subretinal fluid after scleral buckling procedures. *Trans Am Ophthalmol Soc* 1978;76:557–583.

Rubin ML: The induction of refractive errors by retinal detachment surgery. *Trans Am Ophthalmol Soc* 1976;73:452–490.

Ryan SJ, Goldberg MF: Anterior segment ischemia following scleral buckling in sickle cell hemoglobinopathy. *Am J Ophthalmol* 1971; 72:35–50.

Ryan SJ Jr: Cystoid maculopathy in phakic retinal detachment procedures. *Am J Ophthalmol* 1973;76:519–522.

Topilow HW, Ackerman AL: Massive exudative retinal and choroidal detachments following scleral buckling surgery. *Ophthalmology* 1983;90:143–147.

Wilkinson CP, Bradford RH Jr: Complications of draining subretinal fluid. *Retina* 1984;4:1–4.

Wilson, DJ, Green WR: Histopathologic study of the effect of retinal detachment surgery on 49 eyes obtained post mortem. *Am J Ophthalmol* 1987;103:167–179.

CHAPTER 9

Results of Reattachment Surgery

The primary goal of the retinal surgeon is to reattach the retina with the least possible trauma. Surgical cure has been defined as reattachment of the retina for a minimum of 6 months. This is usually accomplished with one operation, but reoperations are occasionally required for a permanent cure.

Between 1968 and 1975, a total of 1101 patients with rhegmatogenous retinal detachment were examined by one of the authors (G.F.H.): 74 were not operated on because 37 had been referred for an opinion only, 31 were thought to be inoperable by scleral buckling, 5 refused surgery, and 1 died preoperatively. Incomplete followup resulted in dropping an additional 27 cases from the series, each of which had retinal attachment when last seen but could not be followed for a full 6 months. All eyes that were detached when last seen were included in the series, even when there had been less than 6 months followup, and they were counted as surgical failures. Results of the remaining 1000 cases are shown in the tables of this chapter. These data are typical of the results reported by various retinal centers.

9-1

RESULTS OF SCLERAL BUCKLING

Approximately 84% of the eyes were reattached with one operation, and reoperations brought the overall cure rate up to 91.3% (Table 9-1). The latter figure includes many types of retinal detachment. These results could be improved by reoperation with vitrectomy techniques in selected cases.

A more accurate prognosis can be determined by reference to specific types of detachment (Table 9-2). Among eight particularly difficult types, the cure rate was significantly reduced when there were gi-

TABLE 9-1

Results of Scleral Buckling (1000 Eyes)

Number of Operations	Percentage Reattached
1	84.1
2	6.5
3	0.7
	91.3

TABLE 9-2

Results of Scleral Buckling in Selected Problem Cases (1000 Eyes)

Preoperative Problem	Incidence (Percentage)*	Number Reattached	Percentage Reattached	Percentage Reattached†
Direct ocular trauma	7.1	60	85	82
Aphakia	36.0	314	87	94
No apparent breaks	9.1	77	85	85
Giant breaks	2.0	14	70	78
PVR, Grade C-1 or less	6.3	50	79	79
PVR, Grade C-2 or more	5.9	25	42	—
Previous retinal surgery elsewhere	8.3	61	73	90
Vitreous hemorrhage	14.5	129	89	89
None of above	47.4	465	98	98

**Several eyes fall into two or more problem categories.*

†Excluding 59 eyes with preoperative PVR, Grade C-2 or worse.

ant breaks, proliferative vitreoretinopathy (PVR), or previous retinal surgery elsewhere. In the series, 59 were referred with PVR, Grade C-2 or worse. Excluding those from the series, there was a cure rate of at least 90% in detachments with aphakia or previous retinal surgery elsewhere. The major obstacle to anatomic cure was PVR. Breaks were defined as giant when they exceeded 90° in size and at least half of the break was above the horizontal meridian. Only 70% were cured. This figure does not include inferior giant breaks, which had a 100% cure rate.

Note that 474 of the eyes did not have any of the eight preoperative problems (see Table 9-2). This group achieved a cure rate of 98%. This "good" prognosis group still included such preoperative findings as corneal scars, miosis, cataract, old detachments, staphylomas, total detachments, retrolental fibroplasia, associated retinoschisis, uveitis, glaucoma, large breaks less than 90°, macular breaks, and coexistent choroidal detachments.

Table 9-3 shows the causes of failure of the first operation, and again the major problem is either preoperative or postoperative PVR. Failures due to inadequately treated breaks responded readily to reoperation. The final causes of failure, despite reoperations, are shown in Table 9-4.

The ultimate goal in retinal surgery is the preservation or restoration of vision. That visual results are generally less satisfactory than anatomic results represents a major challenge for the future.

As shown in Table 9-5, 55% of all the reattached eyes achieved visual acuity of 20/50 or better within 6 months postoperatively. However, 16% were 20/400 or

TABLE 9-3

*Causes of Failure of First Scleral Buckling Operation (1000 Eyes)**

Cause	Percentage
Persistence of preoperative PVR	3.7
Postoperative PVR	5.3
Missed break	1.0
New break	2.1
Leaking anterior to break	0.7
Leaking posterior to break	1.2
Massive vitreous hemorrhage	0.1
Phthisis bulbi	0.1
Unknown	0.9

**Several cases are listed under two or more causes.*

TABLE 9-4

*Causes of Failure of Last Scleral Buckling Operation (1000 Eyes)**

Cause	Percentage
Persistence of preoperative PVR	3.7
Postoperative PVR	4.7
Phthisis bulbi	0.1
Massive vitreous hemorrhage (vitrectomy not available)	0.1
Missed break (refused reoperation)	0.1

**Excluding vitreous surgery.*

TABLE 9-5

Visual Acuity After Scleral Buckling, All Reattached Eyes

Visual Acuity	Number	Percentage
20/20–20/50	499	55
20/60–20/200	263	29
20/400 or worse	151	16
	913	100

TABLE 9-6

*Visual Acuity After Scleral Buckling, All Reattached Eyes Having History of Normal Vision Until Detachment of Fovea**

Visual Acuity	Number	Percentage
20/20–30/50	195	38
20/60–20/200	198	39
20/400 or worse	117	23
	510	100

**Eliminating all cases of amblyopia, macular degeneration, cataract, etc.*

worse. The table includes all eyes, with or without detachment of the macula.

If the macula was included in the detachment, postoperative acuity was generally reduced. There were 510 eyes that had had normal vision before the detachment, then suffered detachment that included the fovea; 38% of these achieved visual acuity of 20/50 or better (Table 9-6).

Of great concern is the group having peripheral detachments with normal macular function: 90% of these retained visual acuity of 20/30 or better, but in the remaining 10% the price for anatomic cure of the peripheral detachment was some decrease in central acuity (Table 9-7).

9-2

RESULTS OF PNEUMATIC RETINOPEXY

Second only to scleral buckling, pneumatic retinopexy is frequently performed for the management of primary retinal detachments. A survey of Retina and Vitreous Societies revealed that 87% of 308 respondents utilized pneumatic retinopexy, performing more than 5000 operations in 1 year. However, another poll of members of these societies revealed that less than half would want the procedure performed on their own eyes. The results of pneumatic retinopexy are presented in Tables 9-8 and 9-9.

A major concern is postoperative new retinal breaks. The multicenter clinical trial revealed that 96% of eyes with new postoperative breaks were successfully reattached. Approximately half of such breaks were managed in the outpatient department without scleral buckling.

TABLE 9-7

Visual Acuity After Scleral Buckling, All Eyes With Preoperative Visual Acuity 20/30 or Better

Visual Acuity	Number	Percentage
20/30 or better	192	90
20/40–20/60	11	5
20/70–20/200	9	4
20/400	2	1
	214	100

TABLE 9-8

Anatomic Results of Pneumatic Retinopexy (103 Eyes)

Procedure	Number	Percentage
Reattached with pneumatic retinopexy*	90	87.4
Failures cured with scleral buckling	11	10.6
Failure cured with vitrectomy	1	1.0
Total eyes reattached	102	99.0

**15 of these eyes received supplemental gas/cryo/laser postoperatively.*

Source: Tornambe PE, Hilton GF, Retinal Detachment Study Group: Pneumatic retinopexy: a multicenter randomized controlled clinical trial comparing pneumatic retinopexy and scleral buckling. Ophthalmology *1989; 96:772–783.*

TABLE 9-9

*Visual Results of 20/50 or Better in Eyes With Macular Detachment for 14 Days or Less (198 Eyes)**

Procedure	Percentage
Pneumatic retinopexy	80
Scleral buckling	56

*$p = 0.01$. *There was no statistically significant difference in the preoperative visual acuity of the two groups. The visual results were not significantly different in the two treatment groups for eyes without preoperative detachment of the macula.*

Source: Tornambe PE, Hilton GF, Retinal Detachment Study Group: Pneumatic retinopexy: a multicenter randomized controlled clinical trial comparing pneumatic retinopexy and scleral buckling. Ophthalmology *1989; 96:772–783.*

SUGGESTED READINGS

Burton TC: Preoperative factors influencing anatomic success rates following retinal detachment surgery. *Trans Am Acad Ophthalmol Otolaryngol* 1977;83:OP499–505.

Burton TC: Recovery of visual acuity after retinal detachment involving the macula. *Trans Am Ophthalmol Soc* 1982;80:475–497.

Escoffery RF, Olk RJ, Grand MG, et al: Vitrectomy without scleral buckling for primary rhegmatogenous retinal detachment. *Am J Ophthalmol* 1985;99:275–281.

Freeman HM, Cox MS, Schepens CL: Traumatic retinal detachments. *Int Ophthalmol Clin* 1974;14:151–170.

Griffith RD, Ryan EA, Hilton GF: Primary retinal detachments without apparent breaks. *Am J Ophthalmol* 1976;81:420–427.

Grizzard WS, Hilton GF: Scleral buckling for retinal detachments complicated by periretinal proliferation. *Arch Ophthalmol* 1982;100: 419–422.

Grizzard WS, Hilton GF, Hammer ME, Taren D: A multivariate analysis of anatomic success of retinal detachments treated with scleral buckling. *Graefe's Arch Clin Exp Ophthalmol* 1994;232:1–7.

Hagler WS, Woldoff HS: Retinal detachment in relation to senile retinoschisis. *Trans Am Acad Ophthalmol Otolaryngol* 1973;77:OP99–113.

Hilton GF, Kelly NE, Salzano TC, et al: Pneumatic retinopexy: a collaborative report of the first 100 operations. *Ophthalmology* 1987; 94:307–314.

Hilton GF, Tornambe PE, Retinal Detachment Study Group: Pneumatic retinopexy: an analysis of intraoperative and postoperative complications [including anatomic results in 1274 eyes]. *Retina* 1991;11:285–294.

Lincoff H, Kreissig I, Richard G, et al: A multicenter trial of the balloon buckle. *Int Congr Ophthalmol* 1982;1:517–519.

Tani P, Robertson DM, Langworthy A: Prognosis for central vision and anatomic reattachment in rhegmatogenous retinal detachment with macula detached. *Am J Ophthalmol* 1981;92:611–620.

Tani P, Robertson DM, Langworthy A: Rhegmatogenous retinal detachment without macular involvement treated with scleral buckling. *Am J Ophthalmol* 1980;90:503–508.

Tornambe PE, Hilton GF, Retinal Detachment Study Group: Pneumatic retinopexy: a multicenter randomized controlled clinical trial comparing pneumatic retinopexy and scleral buckling. *Ophthalmology* 1989;96:772–783.

APPENDIX

*The Technique of Binocular Indirect Ophthalmoscopy**

Morton L. Rosenthal, MD
Seymour Fradin, MD

INTRODUCTION

There is no doubt that binocular, stereoscopic indirect ophthalmoscopy is one of the most important diagnostic methods that we have available. It is absolutely essential for a detailed, panoramic, and complete examination of the fundus.

Still, there are thousands of good ophthalmologists throughout the world who do not master this technique. This is not due to lack of interest or efficiency on their parts. Only a few years ago did Schepens perfect his self-luminous binocular indirect ophthalmoscope and the technique for examination with scleral depression, both of which revolutionized our appreciation of fundus pathology.

The ophthalmologist who was not constantly exposed to this method in his early years of training has all reason to find it difficult and to become impatient with it during his first attempts to use it. Not many have the facility of an instructor at hand and, when searching in the literature for a detailed, step-by-step description of the technique, he finds none exists, even though in multiple papers and lectures it is said by recognized authorities that binocular indirect ophthalmoscopy is a must for the diagnosis and understanding of retinal detachment, tumors, and other diseases of the retina.

The acquisition of proficiency in this method of examination is admittedly difficult. It cannot be developed by casual, infrequent attempts to use the instrument without personal instruction or a step-by-

*Reprinted with permission from *Highlights of Ophthalmology* 1966;9:179–257.

step explanation on how to perform it. Such attempts lead only to frustration, self-doubt, or the feeling that the method itself is worthless.

In the following pages, you will find the most practical and detailed explanation of binocular indirect ophthalmoscopy and scleral depression available in the literature today. It is an effort that we have undertaken as a response to hundreds of letters from the readers of *Highlights* requesting that this be undertaken. It has required 2 full years of work. It is an attempt to lead the ophthalmologist to learning the basic skills necessary to proceed to the eventual mastering of this technique. Diligent, personal effort will do the rest. Daily, repeated use of the techniques here described is essential for the fixation of skills, and a minimum of 3 to 4 months of concentrated effort is necessary to acquire even basic competence, as is true of many other skills in our specialty. The rewards for these efforts will be great. Most ophthalmologists who become skilled in binocular indirect ophthalmoscopy find that they come to prefer it to the direct method, except for rare situations. The sense one acquires of the fundus as a complete entity cannot be achieved by any other technique. The self-confidence and satisfaction that the ophthalmologist feels when examining the entire fundus through this method, free of the doubt that he may have missed significant pathologic entities, will be ample reward for the difficulties encountered in the early stages of learning it.

For this most difficult task of presenting in print, like a moving picture, a technique which is dynamic and greatly subjective, we selected Dr Morton Rosenthal as the author and Dr Seymour Fradin as the artist. Besides his unquestionable prestige as one of the best retinal detachment surgeons in the United States, Dr Rosenthal's ability to present this problem clearly and practically during the course on Binocular Indirect Ophthalmoscopy that he gives at the American Academy* every year is also impressive. Dr Fradin, an associate of Dr Rosenthal's at the retina service in the New York Eye and Ear Infirmary, is not only an able ophthalmologist who knows the subject well but is one of the world's best medical artists, having graduated as a medical artist before studying medicine.

We hope that you will find their work as interesting and stimulating as I have found it.

Benjamin F. Boyd, MD, Editor

---

*Instruction courses offered at the Academy's Annual Meeting are listed each year in the Annual Meeting Program.

COMPARISON OF DIRECT WITH INDIRECT OPHTHALMOSCOPY

In 1851 Helmholtz invented the direct ophthalmoscope and became the first man to see the fundus of a living eye. This event was followed in 1852 by Ruete's development of the indirect method of ophthalmoscopy. It is important to consider the advantages and disadvantages of the two techniques. In order to profitably compare the two methods, a brief consideration of their optics is desirable. Figure 1 shows the optical principles of the direct method. Figure 2 illustrates the optics of the indirect method.

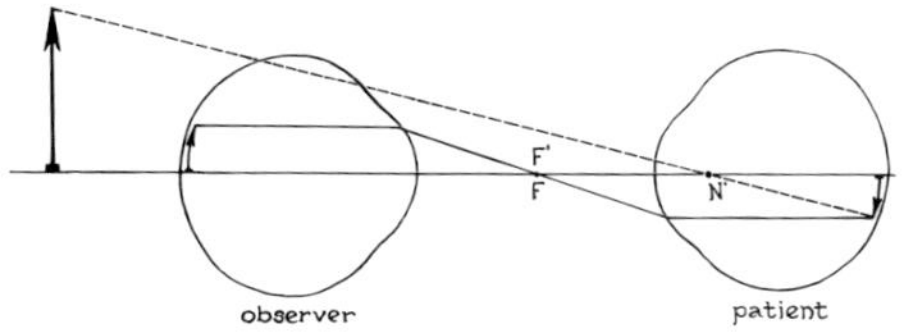

Figure 1 *Optical principles of direct method of ophthalmoscopy.*

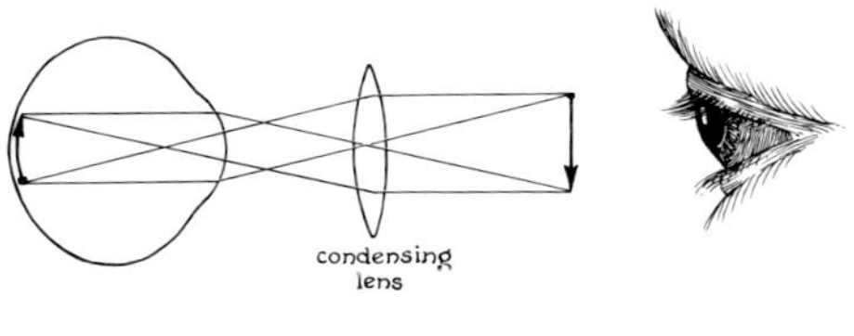

Figure 2 *Optics of indirect ophthalmoscopy.*

The Direct Ophthalmoscopic Image

The image of the fundus obtained with the direct ophthalmoscope is virtual and erect (see Figure 1). The amount of magnification of this image is dependent upon the refractive error of the patient's eye. The magnification in the case of an emmetropic eye is about 15 power. In myopia the magnification is greater, depending upon the degree of myopia, while in hyperopia or aphakia it is less than 15 power.

Each individual field of view permits the visualization of approximately 10° of the fundus in emmetropic eyes. In myopia, the field of view is reduced in proportion to the degree of myopia.

Figure 3A shows what an observer sees in an emmetropic eye, in a single field of view around the disc with direct ophthalmoscopy, in comparison with Figure 3B, which shows the field of view with indirect ophthalmoscopy. Direct ophthalmoscopy permits the study of approximately 60% to 70% of the total fundus area in the emmetropic eye. In aphakia it is sometimes possible to successfully visualize more than this area and, in some cases, to see the ora serrata. In myopia of any significant degree, less than 60% of the fundus may be seen.

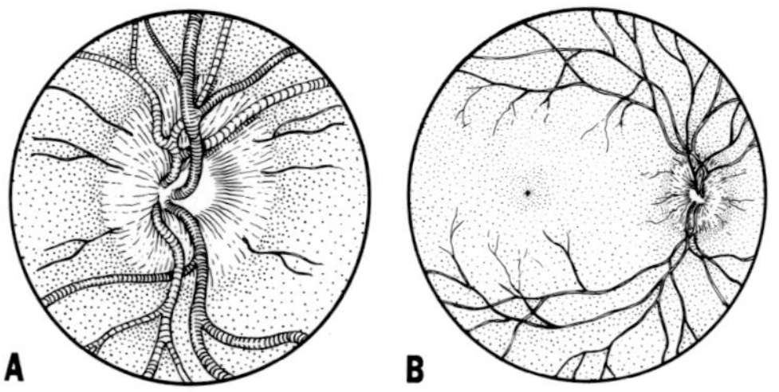

Figure 3 *(A) Shows single field of view in emmetropic eye with direct ophthalmoscope. This field is approximately 10° in diameter. (B) Shows single field of view in same eye seen with indirect ophthalmoscope. This field is approximately 37° in diameter. Since ratio of areas of these fields is proportional to square of radii of fields, it follows that field in part B covers area more than 13 times as great as that in part A. It should be noted that indirect method permits examination of disc, macula, and perimacular retinal vessels at one time. Contrast between these two fields would be even more striking if we assume that eye being examined has 20 D of myopia. In such case, part A would show optic disc occupying entire field of view, while part B would be unchanged. Ratio of areas seen would therefore be much greater than 13 to 1.*

Image brightness is low due to limited output in power. Direct ophthalmoscopes operated by batteries provide about one-half watt of illumination. Instruments operated through transformers deliver several times this amount but never more than several watts.

The image with the usual monocular direct ophthalmoscope is, of course, not stereoscopic.

The working distance of the instrument is only several inches.

The Binocular Indirect Ophthalmoscopic Image

In indirect ophthalmoscopy we examine an inverted, real image. The technique is called indirect because the fundus is seen through a condensing lens. From Figure 2 it can be seen that the image with this method is formed close to the principal focus of the lens, between the lens and the observer. The dioptric power of the condensing lens will determine how close the lens has to be held to the patient's eye in order to produce an image of the fundus. The distance from the observer to the image in front of the lens will depend on the observer's refractive error and whether or not he uses plus lenses in front of his eyes.

The magnification of the image in indirect ophthalmoscopy is little affected by the patient's refractive error but is determined by the power of the condensing lens. For routine use, a 20 D lens is the most satisfactory. Such a lens affords approximately 3.5 power magnification.

The individual ophthalmoscopic fields of view with the 20 D lens will be approximately 37° in diameter (see Figure 3B).

The entire fundus area, including the ora serrata and part of the pars plana of the ciliary body, can usually be examined with this method using scleral depression.

The image is usually stereoscopic, except in cases where the patient's pupil is small.

Modern binocular indirect ophthalmoscopes deliver 18 watts of output, which provide bright fundus images.

CLINICAL COMPARISON OF DIRECT WITH INDIRECT OPHTHALMOSCOPY

The clinical differences between the two methods derive from the differences in optics. The simple statement of those differences in optics, however, cannot begin to describe the range of clinical differences. We shall compare the two techniques with respect to the following considerations:

1. Magnification and illumination (resolution)
2. Field size
3. Stereopsis and depth of focus
4. Effect of opacities in the media of the eye
5. Value of the methods in myopia and other ametropias
6. Study of the equator and far periphery of the eye
7. Use in children and uncooperative adults
8. Fundus drawing
9. Use in the operating room

Magnification and Illumination (Resolution)

The Visualization of Detail The most important clinical characteristics of the image of direct ophthalmoscopy are its high magnification and relatively low brightness. The combination of bright illumination and low magnification results in great resolving power for the indirect system.

Considerable confusion exists on the question of the difference between magnification and resolution and their relative importance in ophthalmoscopy. It has been alleged, for example, that the low magnification of the indirect system precludes the adequate appreciation of fine details in the fundus, particularly vessel details. In reality, the visualization of detail that any optical system permits is a function of its resolving power and not its magnification.

Resolution is defined as the ability of an optical system to separate two points (permit appreciation as separate points) at a standard distance apart. The closer together the two points are, the better the resolving power of the instrument must be in order to permit their being seen as two separate points.

This ability in optical systems is a function of the light available at the points to be resolved, and of the quality of the optical components of the system. It has nothing to do directly with magnification. An image formed by a system that has high resolving power can be magnified more than an image seen through a system of low resolving power. Too much magnifica-

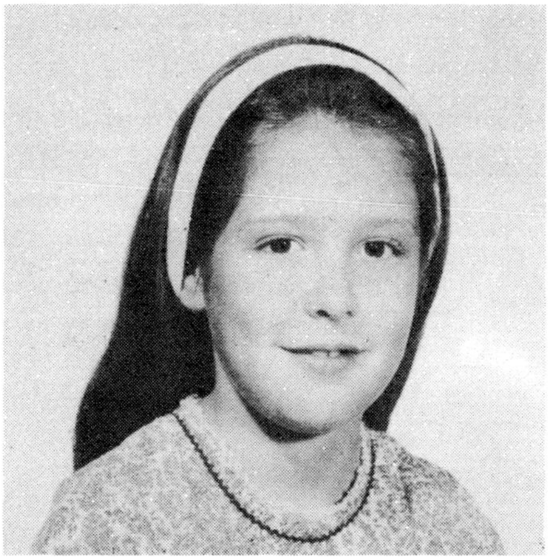

Figure 4 *Halftone reproduction of drawing of child. Detail shown is acceptable at this magnification. Lid margin, iris, and sclera can be seen. If attempt is made to magnify picture to study details in eye, details become unrecognizable, as shown in Figure 5.*

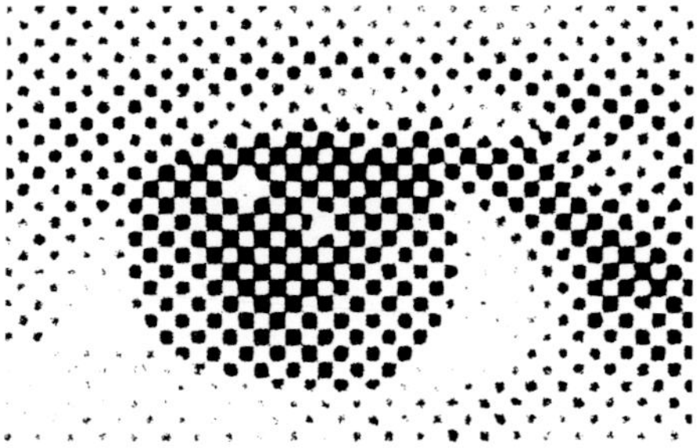

Figure 5 *Enlargement of area of eye of child shown in previous figure. At this magnification, there is less detail visible than at lower magnification of Figure 4.*

tion of a poorly resolved image results in a loss of detail.

A familiar example of this apparent paradox can be found in the common type of photograph seen in newspapers. These pictures are copied by the "halftone" process, which uses screens of various mesh densities to reproduce photographs. The resulting picture consists of a pattern of dots which vary in intensity over different areas of the picture. The picture has acceptable detail when viewed with the naked eye. If one examines such a photographic reproduction of a person's face in a newspaper, there is no difficulty in recognizing the person and even appreciating considerable detail in the face. However, if an attempt is made to examine the image with a magnifying glass to see, for example, the lashes on the lids, then the whole image breaks down into its component dots and even the face is no longer recognizable. The amount of detail inherent in the halftone image simply is not enough to permit magnification without loss of information (Figures 4, 5). In other words, the resolving power of the process is limited.

The halftone example is analogous to our familiar problem in fundus examination with the direct method. The amount of light available at the retinal area being examined determines the degree of magnification that will give useful information. Further magnification only results in a dimmer, blurred (even though larger) image.

It is often difficult for the ophthalmologist to accept this idea in practice although he may recognize it in theory. Most practitioners, when faced with a view of a lesion which is blurred or difficult to interpret, will instinctively seek higher magnification, while the solution for a clearer image is greater resolution, either through greater illumination, lower magnification, or both.

The concepts expressed previously do not imply that magnification is never useful. Frequently, at the posterior pole of the eye the evaluation of fine detail on the disc or in the macula is aided by magnification greater than the 3.5 power obtained with the use of a 20 D condensing lens. The use of greater magnification, however, is contingent on good illumination. For ordinary purposes 3.5 power magnification with excellent illumination, as obtained with the binocular indirect ophthalmoscope, is more than enough to allow an experienced observer to detect minute changes in vessel caliber and to observe details as small as an embolus in a retinal vessel.

During the early stages of learning indirect ophthalmoscopy, it is essential to accept that one has to work with a smaller image size; after a time, one ceases to be troubled by it. After enough experience with indirect ophthalmoscopy, one is rarely aided in an evaluation of detail by increased magnification.

Field Size

The field of view in an emmetropic eye using the direct method is 10°. With the indirect method, using a 20 D condensing lens, the field is 37°. The area seen with the indirect system, in any one field, is 10 times as great. This fact permits the entire fundus to be seen in fewer fields with the indirect method. Most important, indirect ophthalmoscopy permits an appreciation of fundus topography that cannot be obtained with the direct method.

In cases of retinal detachment, for example, where the retina is drawn into folds, the topography of the fundus becomes greatly complex, and the view with the direct ophthalmoscope is difficult to interpret. The image magnification is so great that one sees only a small part of the convoluted retina in any one field, and it is difficult to relate each separate view to adjacent areas.

An analogy can be drawn between the situation of the observer of such a detachment and a mouse on a blanket with many folds. The mouse lies at the bottom of a deep valley formed by two folds in the blanket. He has a clear view only of the blanket he is lying directly on and, since he is very close to it, he can appreciate fine details of the texture of the material. His view of the blanket as a whole, however, is circumscribed by the mountainous folds on either side of him. He cannot know whether his immediate area is typical of the entire blanket or, indeed, if anything at all exists beyond the mountains.

If the mouse is raised from the surface of the blanket several feet, he can now see the entire surface. Then he can see that the little valley he lay in was perhaps a small and insignificant portion of the entire blanket.

Indirect ophthalmoscopy permits the observer to step back from the details of the fundus enough to obtain an appreciation of the detachment as a whole (Figure 6).

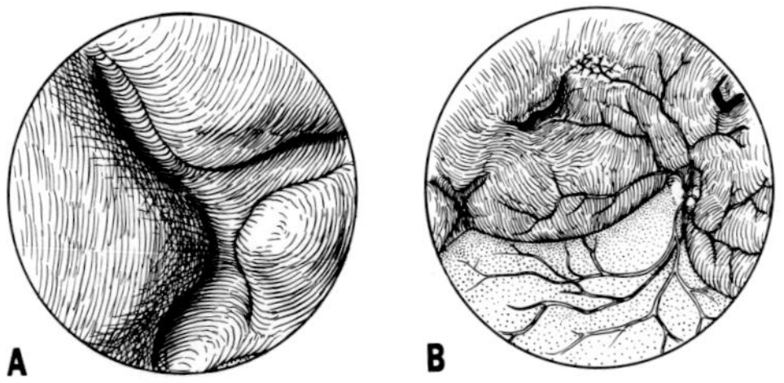

Figure 6 *(A) Shows area of retinal detachment as seen in single ophthalmoscopic field with direct ophthalmoscope. Lesion seen is early star-shaped fold. (B) Shows much larger area of same fundus seen in condensing lens with indirect ophthalmoscope. In latter view, one can see that detachment involves superior retina and includes macular area. Horseshoe-shaped tear is seen at 2-o'clock position posterior to equator, and area of lattice degeneration of retina is noted extending from 10- to 12-o'clock position with large retinal break along its posterior border. Star-shaped fold at 9-o'clock position is seen in its proper relationship to other features of fundus. It would be difficult to draw fundus picture as seen in part B with magnification and smaller field used to visualize part A.*

Other lesions that occupy large areas in the fundus, such as circinate retinopathy of large patches of lattice equatorial degeneration, are rarely appreciated in their true form by direct ophthalmoscopy.

With direct ophthalmoscopy, one sees small parts of these lesions and has to mentally extrapolate the true total picture. With the indirect ophthalmoscope, one sees the entire lesion as a whole and then proceeds to an analysis of the smaller details.

In relating fundus lesions such as retinal holes or tears to other fixed landmarks in the fundus, it is essential to have this overall topographic view in order to make a fundus drawing in which the proper relationships are accurately portrayed.

Stereopsis and Depth of Focus

Monocular direct ophthalmoscopy provides no stereopsis and essentially no depth of focus. Binocular indirect ophthalmoscopy, on the other hand, provides excellent stereopsis and great depth of focus. These qualities of the image are invaluable in the interpretation of masses, folds, and excavations in the fundus. The depth of focus of the system permits the examiner to see the top of a mass in the fundus at the same time that the base is in focus. This is essential during surgical procedures on the retina, such as scleral buckling operations, which produce tumor-like masses whose shape and size require critical evaluation.

This point can be clarified by considering the well-known problem of differentiating a malignant melanoma from a choroidal detachment or choroidal hemorrhage.

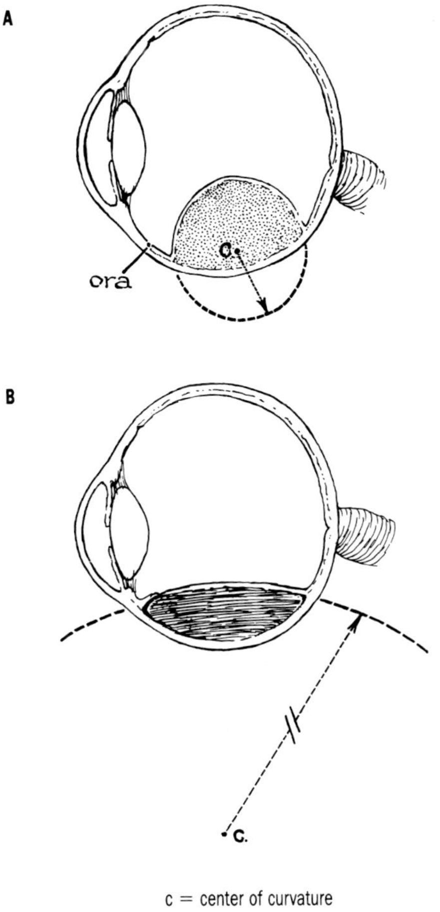

Figure 7 *(A) Shows malignant melanoma of choroid. Tumor is drawn in black. Its form may be considered to be result of intersection of two spheres, the larger of which is eye. Center of smaller sphere is located within eye. Tumor therefore has base that is smaller than its largest diameter. Moreover, unless tumor originates in ciliary body, area of fundus is free of tumor between its base and ora serrata. Spheric shape of tumor results from fact that mass starts from few cells and enlarges by cellular multiplication. "Overhang" of tumor that results from base being smaller than equator of mass is easily appreciated with large field of view of indirect ophthalmoscope and is feature of small tumors. (B) Represents eye containing choroidal hemorrhage or detachment, again shown in black. Form of these lesions may be considered to result from intersection of large imaginary sphere with smaller sphere (eye). Center of larger sphere is outside eye. Since these lesions are caused by extravasation of fluid or blood into choroid, lesion extends rapidly under ciliary body. This elevates ora serrata and makes it easily visible without scleral depression. There is never area between "edge" of choroidal detachment and ora serrata that is uninvolved as is case with tumors. Only structures that choroidal detachments do not dissect into choroid are vortex veins. Choroidal detachments only begin to develop "overhangs" when they become enormous, that is, when they occupy perhaps one third of vitreous cavity.*

These diagnostic criteria are emphasized because they are so easily appreciated by indirect method of ophthalmoscopy and so difficult to appreciate with direct. Differential diagnosis between these lesions almost never presents any difficulty to skilled indirect ophthalmoscopist.

Figure 7 illustrates some important morphologic differences between these lesions that are readily apparent with indirect, but difficult or impossible to appreciate with direct, ophthalmoscopy.

Tumors of the choroid which cause secondary retinal detachment usually cannot be detected by direct ophthalmoscopy, because a detached retina is opaque with this method of examination. This is true for the reasons described previously. Binocular indirect ophthalmoscopy permits a view of the tumor behind the retina, since a detached retina is transparent with the indirect method due to the greater light available.

Opacities in the Ocular Media

Opacities in the ocular media of the patient's eye, either in the cornea, lens, or vitreous, tend to interfere with good resolution of the fundus image by decreasing the light available at the retina. These opacities have a more deleterious effect on the image seen through direct ophthalmoscopy, because the resolution of this system is already marginal.

With the indirect method, examination of the fundus when opacities in the ocular media are present is possible in many cases, even in the presence of marked cataractous lens changes or corneal or vitreous opacities. Such possibility is one of the most gratifying uses of this technique. The surgeon can frequently rule out the presence of retinopathy or alterations in the macula in an eye in which cataract surgery seems indicated but where the history gives little clue to the state of the retina.

On the other hand, macular degeneration may be detected when it is the primary cause of visual loss, perhaps contraindicating lens extraction or at least making the surgeon realistic about the visual prognosis. Such judgments are frequently impossible using direct ophthalmoscopy.

Myopia and Other Ametropias

As has been previously mentioned, with the direct method, the greater the degree of myopia the higher the magnification of the fundus image and the smaller the field of view. When the myopia approaches 20 D or more, it becomes impossible to derive any useful information from direct examination. Yet, it is in precisely such high myopic eyes, with their greater incidence of retinal detachment and macular degeneration, that critical examination is important. Here, indirect ophthalmoscopy is vastly superior, permitting a clear fundus view in spite of refractive error. High cylindric errors strongly and adversely affect the image of direct ophthalmoscopy. This occurs because the high magnification of the system also magnifies the effects of refractive errors on the image.

With the indirect method, the lower magnification minimizes this effect. Furthermore, the condensing lens can be tilted slightly to overcome astigmatic aberrations.

Study of the Equator and Far Periphery of the Eye

The equatorial region of the fundus, seen by direct ophthalmoscopy as an indistinct, blurred area in which little detail can be appreciated, can be readily studied by the indirect method. The reason for this difference lies in the fact that, in order for the equator to be visible, light must travel obliquely through the cornea, lens, and vitreous. This introduces cylindric aberrations in the image, and also increases the number of opacities that the light must encounter between source and image. Direct ophthalmoscopy, by magnifying the image excessively, intensifies the effect of these errors and results in an indistinct picture. The lower magnification of the indirect system permits better resolution.

In addition, the binocular instrument, mounted on the examiner's head, frees one of his hands and permits the accurate use of scleral depression. This technique permits "palpation of the fundus" (Brockhurst) and allows critical study of the equator and the area of the fundus anterior to it, including the ora serrata and the pars plana.

Since 30% of the retina lies anterior to the equator, failure to study this region will result in overlooking serious pathology in many cases. Some diseases such as senile retinal schisis, peripheral uveitis, and some retinal tears defy evaluation by any other technique. The retina anterior to the equator cannot be visualized with the direct ophthalmoscope.

Indirect ophthalmoscopy and scleral depression are of particular value in differentiating retinal breaks from retinal hemorrhages (see Figure 38), in recognizing a raised from a depressed lesion, and in detecting whether a hemorrhage or foreign body lies on or anterior to the retina (Figure 8).

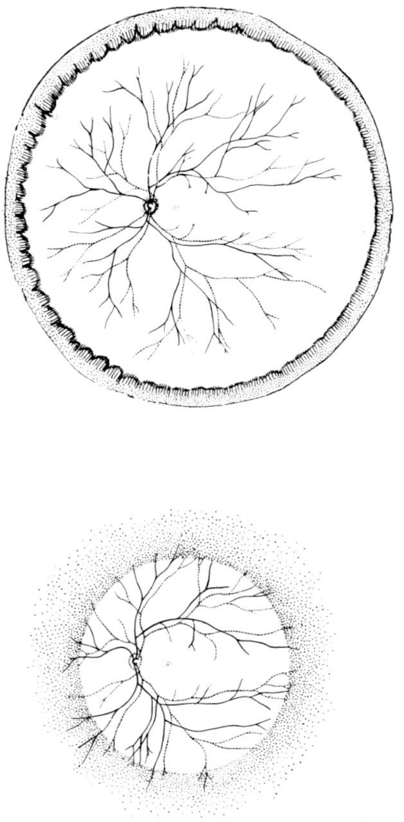

A

B

Figure 8 *(A) Shows area of fundus accessible to view by indirect ophthalmoscopy and scleral depression: all of retina and posterior one third of pars plana. (B) Shows how much of same fundus is visible by direct ophthalmoscopy: only about 70% of total fundus area.*

Children and Uncooperative Adults

With uncooperative young children and disoriented adults, or those with nystagmus, it is often not possible to examine the fundus with the direct method. With indirect, since the field of view is so much larger, even a wildly gyrating disc can usually be observed satisfactorily. Moreover, since the examiner can rapidly shift his attention from one eye to the other, a quick and accurate comparison of two eyes can be made. Children generally react favorably to the more impersonal distance of indirect examination.

Fundus Drawing

Modern techniques of retinal surgery depend to a great extent on the accurate drawing of the fundus. Considerable attention will be given to this later. A large field of view is essential to ease in moving from one area of the fundus to the next, which, in turn, is essential for adequate perspective in making a drawing of the fundus. Direct ophthalmoscopy is totally inadequate to this need. The examiner attempting to draw a fundus using direct ophthalmoscopy, particularly if examining a myopic eye, is in an analogous position to a man with severe concentric contraction of his field due to retinitis pigmentosa trying to paint a mural.

Use in the Operating Room

During surgery the ophthalmologist faces some of the most severe demands on ophthalmoscopic technique that he could encounter. In the first place, the fundus to be examined is usually a difficult one, such as a retinal detachment. Furthermore, during the course of surgery the cornea may become hazy or abraded. Finally, the fundus picture may change rapidly or frequently, as is the case in the later stages of a retinal operation. This requires rapid and accurate evaluation to permit the operator to plan the next maneuver. Direct ophthalmoscopy is, in all respects, inadequate in such situations. A complex fundus picture, particularly one which is frequently changing, requires too much time for evaluation with direct ophthalmoscopy; this is unsatisfactory. A corneal abrasion that might present no hindrance to clear view with the indirect method might prove an insurmountable problem to direct ophthalmoscopy.

The close working distance of the direct instrument invites contamination of the field. With the indirect method, the lens is kept sterile and less danger of contamination is present.

Most important of all considerations, however, is that the indirect method permits accurate localization of all retinal breaks and other fundus landmarks by the scleral depression technique under direct observation by the surgeon. With it, the guesswork is eliminated from the localization procedure.

Binocular indirect ophthalmoscopy also permits the accurate removal of intraocular foreign bodies when the media are not opaque and a more precise diagnosis and treatment of choroidal or retinal tumors.

PROBLEMS IN LEARNING INDIRECT OPHTHALMOSCOPY

In learning the technique of indirect ophthalmoscopy, a number of problems present themselves:

1. The patient must be properly prepared and positioned in order to be satisfactorily examined.

2. The instrument itself must be properly adjusted on the examiner's head.

3. A technique must be developed for correctly holding the condensing lens and the scleral depressor and for dealing with troublesome light reflexes.

4. The small size of the fundus image in the condensing lens is initially disturbing to someone used to the larger magnification of direct ophthalmoscopy.

5. The inversion of the image is initially confusing.

6. Diplopia may be encountered.

7. Anatomic and pathologic entities differ in their appearance when viewed with the indirect ophthalmoscope as opposed to the direct ophthalmoscope.

From the presently available binocular indirect ophthalmoscopes, the best known as well as most efficient are (1) the instrument manufactured by the American Optical Company, and (2) the instrument manufactured by Keeler. Several other companies have produced instruments that accomplish similar purposes.

Adjusting the Instrument

Essentially, all of these instruments consist of a light source mounted on the head, oculars containing plus power, and prisms to enable the observer to sight down a narrow axis. The eyepieces can be adjusted for individual interpupillary distances. Several screws permit movement of the headpiece on several axes, allowing fine adjustment of the light direction. These details are shown in Figures 9 and 10.

Much of the frustration attendant upon first using the binocular indirect ophthalmoscope can be obviated by carefully adjusting the instrument to one's own head. For those who are not familiar with the use of the instrument, we shall describe the step-by-step procedure of how to adjust it. We will use, merely as an example, the American Optical (AO) ophthalmoscope (Figure 11) because it is the one we are more familiar with, although comments will apply equally to other instruments.

The first adjustment to be made by the examiner should be the headband. The instrument must fit comfortably on the head without undue tightness of the headband. The older model of the AO ophthalmoscope has straps on the upper part of the headband that can be adjusted.

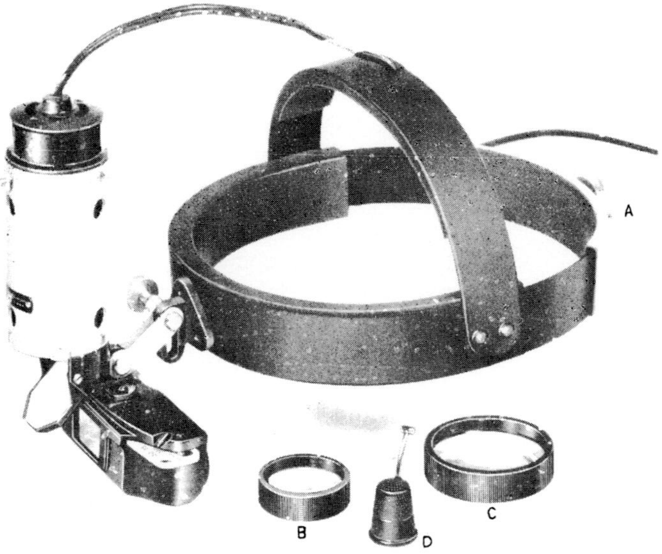

Figure 9 *Basic instrument without accessories. (A) Knob at back of headband is used to tighte band. Strap across top of head is not adjustable in this model. Shown also are lenses supplied with instrument: (B) 30 D aspheric lens, 35 mm in diameter, and (C) 14 D biconvex lens, 50 mm in diameter. It is convenient to supplement these with 35-mm plano-convex 20 D lens for routine use (available from New York Eye and Ear Infirmary Optical Department). (D) Scleral depressor is also shown.*

These should be shortened so that they rest on the head, taking some of the weight of the instrument off the headband. This adjustment must be made for individual head sizes. It is well not to allow other people to use your instrument nor to put it back in the case after using it each time, because such frequent readjustments will cause loosening of the adjusting screws and a generally unsatisfactory fit. Like anything else that one wears habitually, it will tend to fit better as time goes on.

Once the headband fits satisfactorily, we should concern ourselves with the adjustment of the eyepiece. The instrument should be plugged in and the light turned on during this adjustment. We can see in Figure 9 that the light housing and eyepiece are attached to the headband by a double bracket. This bracket is attached

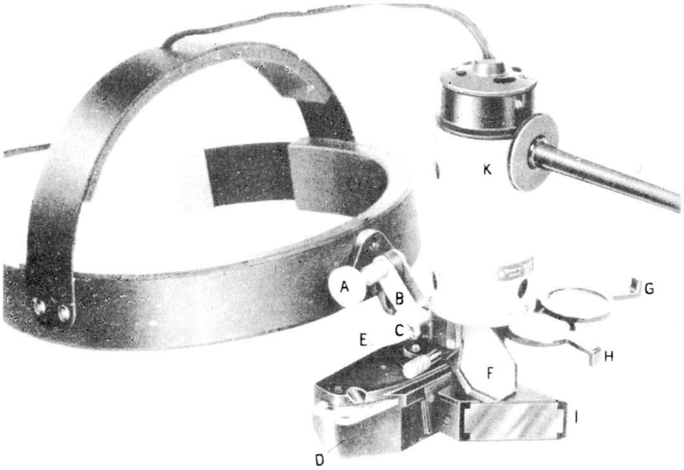

to the headband above by a knurled screw and to the eyepiece below by a slotted nut. These two screws afford movement on their shafts that permit adjustments of the eyepiece toward and away from the examiner's face, while permitting simultaneous adjustment of the angle that the eyepiece makes with the plane of the examiner's face. The knurled-knob adjustment also permits raising and lowering of the eyepieces. The two screws must be kept tight or the eyepiece–light housing will swing freely and rest against the face. A screwdriver of the appropriate size should be kept in the case to permit frequent adjustment. The function of the two screws can be easily demonstrated by moving the eyepiece back and forth and observing all possible movements. One should swing the eyepiece down in front of the examiner's eye until the eyepieces are as close to the pupil as possible, perpendicular to the pupillary axis, and yet not resting on the bridge of the nose.

Figure 10 *View of right side of ophthalmoscope showing (A) knurled knob that connects headband to (B) eyepiece bracket and permits bracket to slide up and down as well as pivot. (C) Lower screw attaching bracket to (D) eyepiece is also shown. This screw is slotted for screwdriver. (E) Thin-knurled shaft just below this screw is adjustment for (F) mirror which controls angle of light beam. Shown are (G) neutral-density and (H) red-free light filters which are optional equipment. They are not of much use. Notice (I) half-silvered mirror which enables another observer to obtain monocular view of field that examiner sees with stereopsis. This is useful for teaching. (J) Removable handle protruding from (K) light housing is supplied with idea that it could be used sterile in operating room. This is of little practical use.*

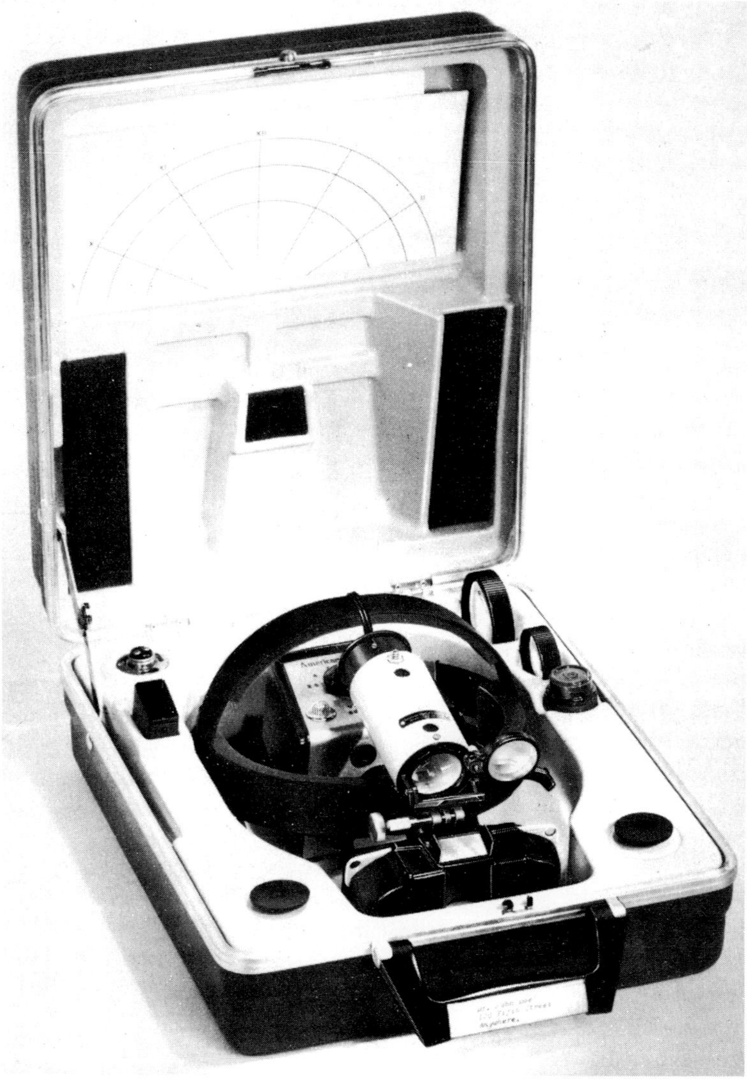

Figure 11 *American Optical instrument in its carrying case.*

This will involve pivoting the eyepiece on both of the pivot screws.

The wearing of spectacles by the examiner makes it difficult to bring the eyepiece of the instrument as close to the eye as is desirable. The closer the eyepiece is to the eye, the larger the field of view and the more satisfactory is the manipulation of the instrument.

The eyepiece of the American Optical instrument has a +2 D lens before each eye. Since the working distance is approximately one third of a meter, this arrangement enables an emmetropic observer to use only 1 D of accommodation to view the image in the condensing lens. Myopes can increase or decrease the plus power to suit their refraction. Presbyopes generally will need the equivalent of an intermediate range add or their addition for near. Hyperopes will need their distance correction added to the +2 D already in the eyepieces.

We should now adjust the interpupillary distance of the oculars. This should be done by loosening the two screws on top of the eyepiece which secure the eyepiece adjustment bars so that these can be easily pushed in or out. With the instrument on the head and the light turned on, the oblong spot of light should be directed at a vertical white surface a full arm's length away from the observer.

The left eye should now be closed and, with the right hand, the right eyepiece adjustment bar is moved in and out until the square of light is exactly centered in the field of the right eye. We are concerned now only with horizontal centering. When the right eyepiece has been adjusted, the right eye is closed and the left eyepiece is adjusted in the same way. With both eyes open, the light is now adjusted vertically by moving the small knurled shaft that controls the mirror until the light occupies the upper half of the field of view.

We should now have a comfortable, single, binocular view of the square of light. It should occupy the upper half of our field, and it should be centered horizontally. Most of the complaints of diplopia that are heard from some beginners who try to use the instrument are due to a failure to make these adjustments accurately. The interpupillary distance should not be adjusted while observing the spot of light at the working distance at which one ordinarily adjusts a binocular loupe, or diplopia will result at the much longer working distance of the binocular ophthalmoscope, and certainly fatigue will be rapid. Interpupillary distance adjustments must be made at an arm's-length working distance.

The sensation of strain from induced phoria due to faulty adjustment of interpupillary distance causes headaches that are falsely attributed to the weight of the instrument. An experienced observer rarely notices the weight of the instrument, even after long periods of use.

If diplopia persists even after careful attention to the above directions, the examiner should have his fusional amplitudes checked and improved with exercises if indicated.

Choice of Condensing Lenses

At present, a confusing assortment of lenses is available to the ophthalmoscopist: he may choose between plano-convex, bi-convex, and aspheric lenses. In addition, claims have been made as to the advantages of aspheric lenses in different powers, which further confuses the issue.

Insofar as the power of the lens is concerned, the lower the power, the greater the magnification and the more limited the individual ophthalmoscopic field. Furthermore, lower-power lenses have to be held farther from the patient's eye, and this makes their use more difficult. About the lowest power that is practical to use in binocular indirect ophthalmoscopy is 13 or 14 D. Lenses of such low power will rarely be used.

The most generally useful power in a condensing lens is about 20 to 22 D. This gives a good compromise between field size and magnification. It permits a convenient working distance from the patient's eye and, in the usual 35-mm diameter, it is easy to grasp.

In this power range of 20 to 22 D, there are available plano-convex, bi-convex, and aspheric lenses to choose from. The significant difference between these various lenses lies in the magnitude of troublesome light reflexes caused by the refracting surfaces.

In general, the more plano a surface is, the more objectionable will be its reflexes when the surface faces the observer. Conversely, the more convex the surface that faces the observer, the less troublesome the reflexes. Thus, a plano-convex lens of 20 D with a plano surface and a +20 surface will give the maximum of troublesome reflexes when the plano surface is facing the ophthalmoscopist and the minimum number of reflexes when the strongly convex side faces him.

In the case of the bi-convex lens with two surfaces of +10 D, either way it is held it will have fewer reflexes than the plano-convex lens held incorrectly with the plano surface toward the observer; however, it will not be as reflex-free as the plano-convex lens that is properly held with the strongly plus surface toward the observer.

There is, therefore, a clear superiority of a plano-convex 20 D spheric lens, properly held, over a biconvex 20 D lens in which each surface is a +10 D lens. The aspheric lens, since it has one strongly convex side, has the same advantages over the biconvex lens. However, in the 20 D power, it has no clinically detectable advantage over the spheric plano-convex lens.

When we try to use lenses of powers greater than 20 D, such as 30 D or 40 D, with the purpose of obtaining less magnification, aspheric lenses are essential. Such lenses, since they give less magnified images, give correspondingly larger fields of view. This is occasionally useful in examining patients with small pupils which dilate poorly or patients with extremely complicated retinal topography.

All lenses used for indirect ophthalmoscopy should have coated surfaces to reduce reflexes.

To summarize the question of choice of condensing lenses:

1. The most generally useful lens is a plano-convex +20 D lens (available from the New York Eye and Ear Infirmary Optical Department), held with the convex side toward the observer. It is clearly superior to a biconvex 20 D lens. It is equal in performance to a 20 D aspheric lens and it costs one fourth the price of a glass aspheric lens. Plastic aspheric lenses are reasonable in price, but they scratch easily.*

2. On occasion, a 30 D or 40 D lens may prove useful. Such a strong lens must be aspheric.

The Preparation of the Patient

The inherent advantages of any method of examination can be negated by inadequate preparation of the patient and by failure to choose a suitable place of examination. A reasonable physician would not attempt to examine the heart in a noisy room. Likewise, it is useless to attempt to do critical indirect ophthalmoscopy in a patient whose pupil is not widely dilated or who is seated in a lighted room.

The first prerequisite for an adequate examination is a patient who has at least some idea of what he should expect in the examination. He should be warned that the light is intense, more so than in any examination he has experienced. He should be reassured that no harm can come to him from this bright light. This is important, since even some intelligent patients are concerned in a vague way that the light may be "too bright."

Pupillary Dilation The pupil should be dilated to the maximum possible diameter. Mydriatics, such as 10% Neo-Synephrine, used alone are totally inadequate; the moment the bright light is projected into the eye, the strong stimulation to sphincter contraction will overcome the action of the dilator muscle, and the pupil will become miotic. On the other hand, cycloplegics used alone, while much more satisfactory than mydriatics alone, do not give maximum dilation. They do, however, result in a dilation that is not affected by the strong light and may be used alone.

The most satisfactory dilation is achieved by the use of any cycloplegic plus 10% Neo-Synephrine drops. This combination produces a wide and lasting result. The choice of a cycloplegic is determined by how long the examiner wishes the pupil to remain dilated and not by how widely he wishes it dilated.

For routine fundus study, Cyclogyl plus Neo-Synephrine, or Cyclomydril alone, is satisfactory. In cases where a retinal detachment or other pathology exists requiring fundus study over a period of days or

---

*The 20 D Nikon condensing lens or its equivalent is discussed in Section 3-9.

weeks, scopolamine 0.25% and 10% Neo-Synephrine have proved to be the best combination. Atropine in such cases carries a greater hazard of skin sensitization if used long enough.

Maximal dilation may be impossible in some eyes due to posterior synechiae, secondary membranes, sphincter damage following round pupil cataract extraction, or other causes. Such patients are not easy subjects for the inexperienced observer to examine. The positioning and the fine movements of the condensing lens become so critical that the examination of such patients should be deferred until some facility with this technique has been achieved. An experienced examiner can see through a miotic pupil but with difficulty.

Medications to Be Avoided Nothing should be put in the eye which might cause corneal hazing. Topical anesthetics such as tetracaine or cocaine often result in epithelial edema and may make the appreciation of fine detail difficult. As in the case of a small pupil, such a situation may present little trouble to the expert but may make accurate positioning of the condensing lens impossible for the novice. Ointments of any kind should not be used, as they make the lids slippery and cause blurring of the image.

Position of the Patient The patient should now be positioned lying flat on a stretcher (Figure 12). The supine position offers such great advantages over the seated one that it should be used in all but a few rare instances. The stretcher should be just high enough to reach the examiner's hips. The patient's head should be unsupported. If any dorsal kyphosis is present, a small flat pillow should be used to prevent hyperextension of the neck and assure comfort. The neck should not be flexed at this stage of the examination, and the table or stretcher should not be tilted up, since this makes examination of some parts of the periphery of the retina difficult (see Figure 12).

First Steps in Seeing the Fundus

Preliminary Steps The patient now lies in a relaxed position. The examiner will have complete control of the patient's head by holding it. He also can control the upper and lower lids and the condensing lens simultaneously. Furthermore, unlike examinations performed with the patient sitting, the examiner does not have to hold the condensing lens out horizontally at arm's length, which is a fatiguing position to hold for more than a few minutes.

The patient should now be asked to look in the cardinal directions of gaze. This serves to alert the examiner to how well the patient can follow such commands. Some patients have poor voluntary control of eye movements. In such cases, it is advisable to have the patient hold out his own hand as a fixation object and look at it (Figure 13). The proprioceptive impulses originating from the arm serve to

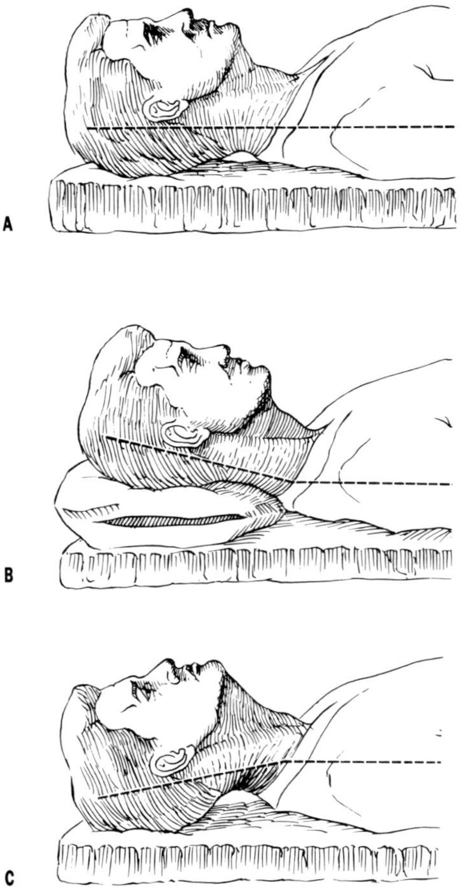

Figure 12 *(A) Correct position of head for beginning examination of fundus. Note that head is neither flexed nor extended; plane of face is horizontal. (B) Position is unsatisfactory for general examination of fundus. It would be difficult with head flexed this much to see inferior periphery. However, sometimes this position of head is useful in aiding visualization of superior periphery. (C) Position is also not good for general examination of fundus. Extension of neck makes examination of superior periphery of fundus difficult because of interference of chin. This position is sometimes useful in examining inferior periphery.*

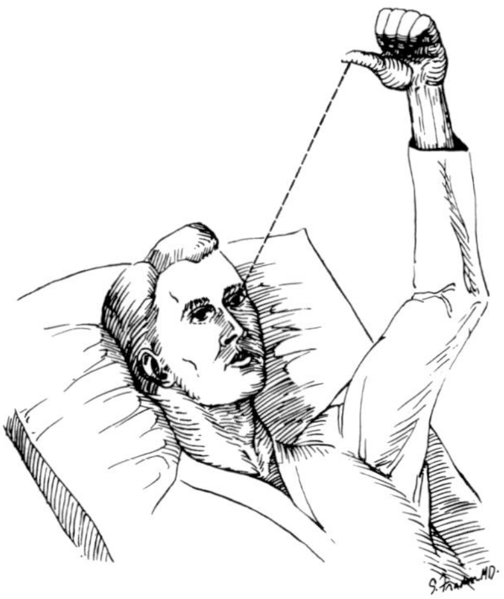

Figure 13 *Use of patient's own hand as target has several advantages over other possible objects. Patient with sight will then use visual stimuli from his hand for fixation in addition to proprioceptive impulses. Latter are important in case of blind, monocular, or uncooperative patients.*

enable even a blind patient to cooperate. The patient must be repeatedly urged to open the fellow eye.

Keeping the Other Eye Open The examiner holds apart the lids of the eye being examined. If the patient closes the other eye, Bell's reflex will cause the examined eye to roll up also. It is useless to have the patient hold the fellow eye open with his hand since this only intensifies the Bell's reflex. Constant reassurance and reminding are necessary to keep the patient from allowing the opposite eye to close. As he becomes more light-adapted, this tendency decreases.

Good cycloplegia is the most important single factor in getting cooperation in this regard. The eye with inadequate cycloplegia is photophobic.

Holding the Condensing Lens With the patient in the proper position on the stretcher and with the ophthalmoscope adjusted as described previously, we are ready to attempt to see the fundus. The problem now arises as to with which hand to hold the condensing lens. The first impulse is to hold it in the hand with which one ordinarily writes. This may make the initial viewing of the fundus easier but will result in difficulties later on when deciding with which hand to hold the scleral depressor. It is advisable to use the writing hand for the scleral depressor and the other hand for holding the lens. This may prove initially awkward but in the long run affords greater facility for examination; it is difficult for most people to use the scleral depressor in the nonwriting hand. Thus, right-handed persons should hold the condensing lens in the left hand and use the scleral depressor with the right. Left-handed persons should, in most cases, use the right hand for the condensing lens and the left for scleral depression. One should consistently use the same hand to hold the lens; otherwise, it will be difficult to develop the reflex skills necessary to do efficient ophthalmoscopy.

Position of the Examiner's Hands The precise manner of holding the condensing lens is of critical importance (Figure 14). It should be grasped between the tip of the flexed index finger and the ball of the extended thumb. The wrist should be flexed moderately and the third, fourth, and fifth fingers should be extended. The extended third finger is used to hold the upper or lower lid of the patient—which lid depends on the side of the patient one is standing on. The thumb of the opposite hand is used to retract the lid not held by the third finger (Figure 15). With the fourth and fifth fingers of the hand which is holding the lens, and with the other hand, the examiner holds the patient's head firmly. The advantages of this position are as follows:

The extended third finger acts as a pivot which enables the observer to tilt the lens in all planes merely by rocking the forearm on the tip of the finger. The lens can be moved with critical control closer to or farther away from the eye (see Figure 14B) by increasing or decreasing the flexion of the index finger. If the lens is incorrectly grasped between the ball of the index finger or the terminal joint of that finger and the ball of the thumb, it is difficult to make the fine adjustments in lens position so essential to critical scanning of the fundus.

To obtain the initial fundus view, the light intensity on the scope should be turned down to one-half maximum output by adjusting the transformer. The light should be directed onto the patient's eye without the condensing lens being in place, to initiate light adaptation. After about 10 or 15 seconds, the patient should be asked to look up so that the light will be thrown onto the superior fundus and away from the macula.

Let us assume that we are about to examine the patient's left eye (see Figure 15). We stand alongside him on the left side and, holding the lens as described, place the extended third finger of the hand which holds the lens on the left lower lid, retracting it. The thumb of the opposite hand (right thumb in this example) grasps the upper lid as indicated. The light is now directed into the pupil, and the lens is interposed about 1 inch from the patient's eye. The examiner must keep the arm which holds the lens extended and keep his head at arm's length from the lens. The lens is now slowly held away from the patient's eye by increasing the flexion of the index finger. When the lens is at a proper distance away, it will fill with the image of the fundus, which should be clear and striking in its stereopsis. No matter how often one may perform this examination, it is impossible not to be struck by the clarity, beauty, and plastic quality of the image of the fundus.

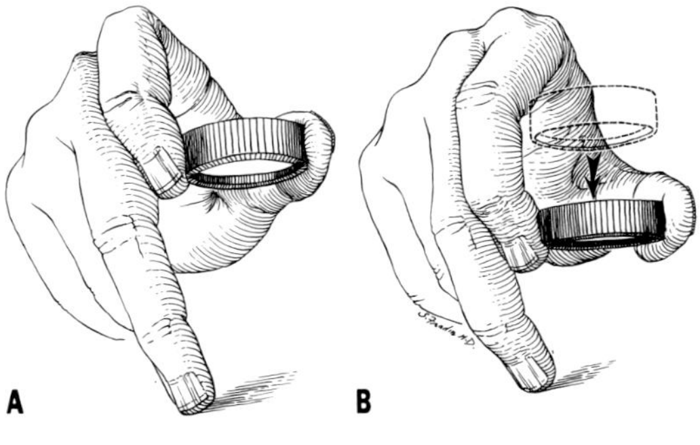

A B

Figure 14 *(A) Lens is grasped between ball of thumb and tip of index finger. Wrist is extended, and third finger is extended as pivot. (B) Manner in which lens is moved closer to or away from eye is shown.*

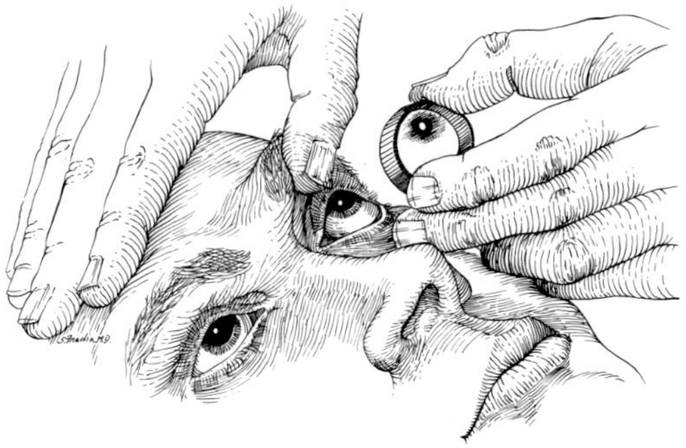

Figure 15 *Examiner is observing superonasal part of patient's fundus. He stands to left of patient, and third finger of left hand controls lower lid. Right hand controls head, and thumb of right hand controls upper lid. To observe temporal half of left fundus, examiner should stand on right side of patient. Left third finger then controls upper lid, and right thumb retracts lower lid.*

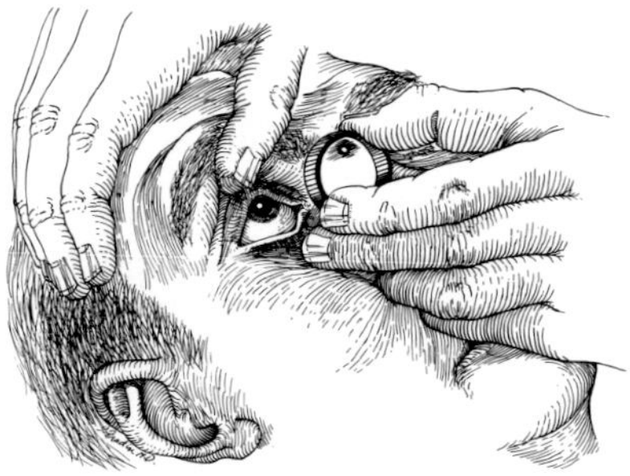

Figure 16 *Observer is standing on left side of patient, examining superior retina, and is shown holding lens in his left hand. Thumb and index finger control lens, and third finger simultaneously retracts lower lid. Right hand is used to control patient's head, and thumb of this hand retracts upper lid. These positions of hands permit examination of entire temporal half of right fundus. To observe nasal half, examiner should stand on right side of patient. Left third finger will now be used to hold upper lid, and right thumb now retracts lower lid. Figure 20 shows this position. Considerable movement of examiner's body and head will be necessary to see entire fundus.*

For examination of the patient's right eye, the same principles are followed, as explained in Figure 16.

Troublesome Reflexes With the fundus now in view, a number of problems become apparent. Reflexes from the condensing lens surface may be troublesome (Figure 17). These reflexes correspond to images of the ophthalmoscope bulb formed by the anterior and posterior condensing lens surfaces. One will note a large anterior reflex and a smaller posterior one (see Figure 17A). These reflexes can be made to move in opposite directions from each other by slightly tilting the lens (see Figures 17B,C). Thus, they can be moved away from the center of the lens so that they do not obscure the object being studied (Figure 18).

Any dirt or fingerprints on the lens surfaces cause great interference with the view of the fundus. Such dirt causes more difficulty in seeing the retina than if it were present in the vitreous. The condensing lens must be kept scrupulously clean and free of fingerprints.

Shifting From One Part of the Fundus to the Next It will now also become evident that small lateral movements of the lens can be made without losing the image of the fundus filling the lens. It will be noted that such movements do not enable you to see another field of view. In fact, if the movements laterally are too great, the image is lost. These fine movements do bring out parallactic movements of objects in the fundus. In order to get from one part of the fundus to the next, more than mere movement of the lens is needed.

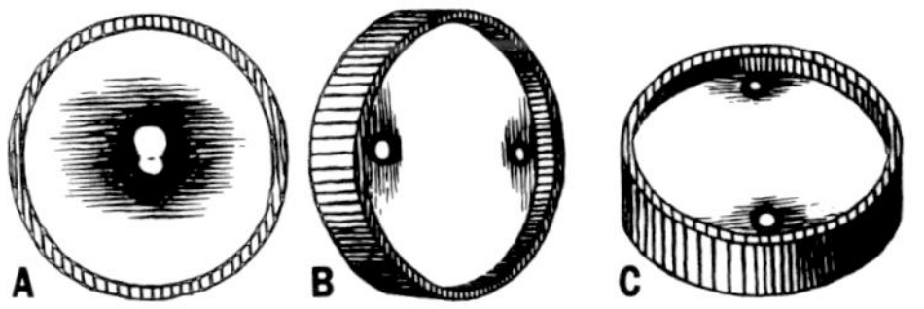

Figure 17 *(A) With condensing lens held perpendicular to visual axis as shown, anterior reflex and smaller posterior reflex are centered in lens, causing maximum interference with vision. (B) Lens has been tilted to left, causing anterior reflex to move to right and posterior to move to left. Observer can look between them. (C) Reflexes can be moved vertically by tilting lens forward. Anterior reflex always moves in direction of lens tilt, and posterior reflex away from it.*

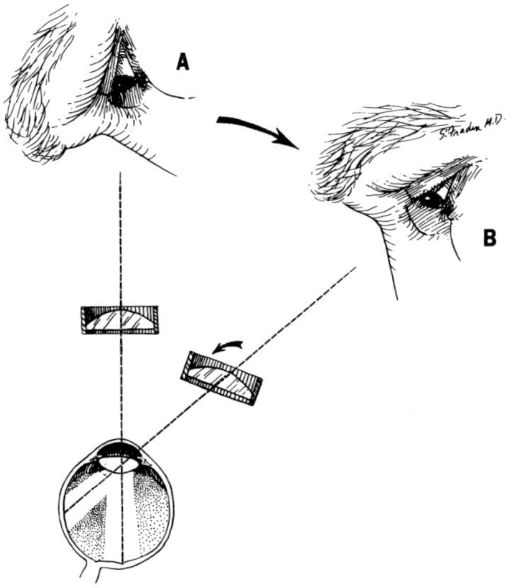

Figure 18 *(A) Shows observer viewing area of macula. Lens is shown perpendicular to visual axis. In this position, light reflexes are superimposed and view of macula is obscured. It is necessary to tilt lens with reference to visual axis. (B) Observer is shown viewing equatorial area of eye. Lens is correctly tilted to eliminate effect of light reflexes. Lens should be tilted at slightly more acute angle to visual axis when observing extreme periphery of eye than when viewing posterior pole to compensate for oblique astigmatism. With experience, this correction is made automatically to clear image.*

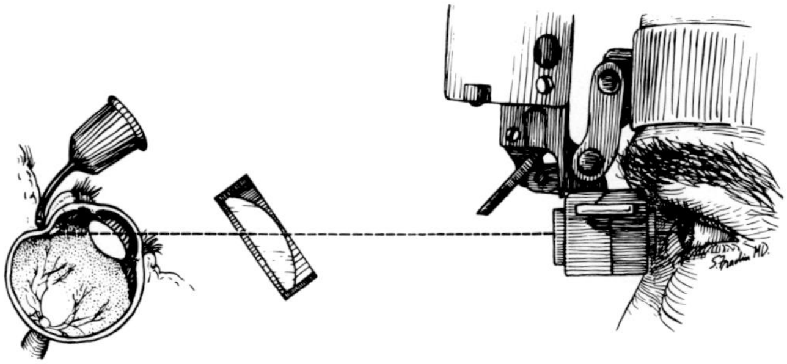

Figure 19 *Alignment of eyepiece, condensing lens, pupil, and fundus area on visual axis.*

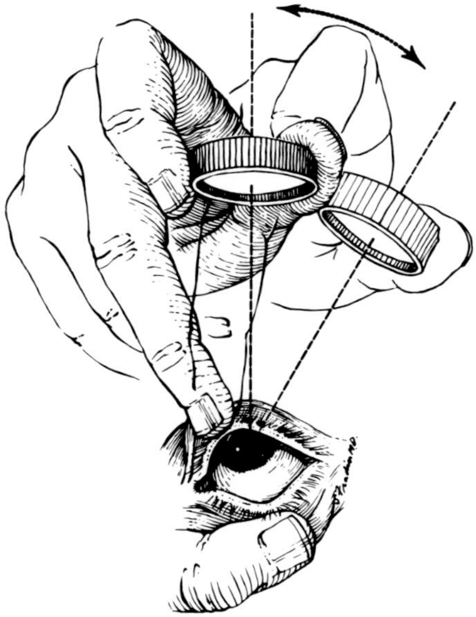

Figure 20 *Previously described technique of holding lens is shown. Importance of extended third finger is apparent, since it is pivot on which precise control of rotation of visual axis must depend. In this instance, same finger holds upper lid open, and thumb of opposite hand holds lower lid.*

We must consider the entire image system as consisting of a number of vital elements arranged on a straight line (Figure 19). These elements are the observer's macula, the eyepiece of the scope, the center of the condensing lens, the patient's pupil, and the object observed in the fundus. All these elements must be kept on a rigid axis or the image is lost. To move from one point in the patient's retina to another, the whole axis must be pivoted like a lever, with the fulcrum or fixed point being the patient's pupil. Thus, the observer must move his head and tilt the lens simultaneously by using the third finger as a pivot. The importance of the proper holding of the lens is now apparent. One must be able to maintain the lens at the correct distance from the patient's eye and still tilt it smoothly in all directions at the same time. To do this, the third finger must be kept rigid (Figure 20).

The coordinated movement of the observer's head and the tilting of the lens is a maneuver that takes considerable practice. The head is not moved on the neck but, rather, the whole torso is moved from side to side and forward and backward while the lens is appropriately tilted (Figure 21). It is essential to practice this maneuver until it is completely natural and automatic.

This is the major stumbling block in learning indirect ophthalmoscopy. Some ophthalmologists never master this step and consequently do not continue to progress from this stage. These persons, in order to see the fundus, will have the patient look in one direction and then observe the fundus field in view. They then have the patient look in another direction and again find the image of the fundus and examine it. This results in seeing only isolated areas of the fundus. Not only is it inevitable to miss large areas of the retina in this way but one cannot ever gain an overall appreciation of fundus topography or remain oriented, and it makes virtually hopeless the task of scleral depression. It is therefore essential that we master the "sweeping" of the fundus. The best exercise to develop facility in this regard is as follows:

The observer should find the posterior pole of the eye and the disc. He should now have in one field of view the disc, macula, and both the superior and inferior temporal vessels. One vessel should be picked out and followed from the disc to as far anterior as can be seen by the observer's movements alone. This vessel should then be followed back to the disc. This should be repeated over and over again until a smooth body–lens coordination is achieved and a continuous, sweeping picture of the fundus can be seen all along the path of the vessel. It may take weeks to acquire this ability but it is useless to go on until this is accomplished.

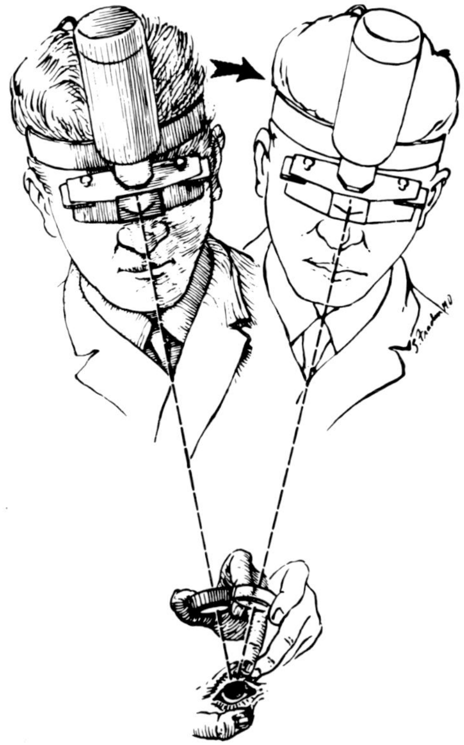

Figure 21 *Axis is formed by examiner's visual axis (split by prisms in headpiece), condensing lens, patient's pupil, and area of fundus under study. Fulcrum of this axis is patient's pupil. In order to observe another part of fundus, observer's head must move and lens tilt in such way that new axis also has its fulcrum in pupil.*

Orientation

The Problem of the Inverted Image Up until now, no mention has been made of a subject that most people consider the major problem in this examination technique, that is, the inverted nature of the image. We have intentionally avoided consideration of this problem until now, since we consider it subordinate to the major one of seeing continuous fundus details. It is only after one has achieved the ability to see the fundus and to follow all vessels easily that any consideration should be given to the inversion of the image. Most, if not all, of the confusion regarding the inverted image has as its basis the constant attempts of the inexperienced examiner to relate the indirect image to his concept of what the direct ophthalmoscopic image should be. We may begin the consideration of this problem by an analogy to learning a new language.

Learning a new language successfully means incorporating the vocabulary, grammar, idioms, and thought into one's own unconscious thinking processes. One must learn to "think" in the new language. It is obvious that if one merely translates the foreign expression and words directly into one's native tongue, a stiff and unsatisfactory grasp of the language results. People who learn a language from a book by relating it constantly to their own language can never think in the new tongue. To achieve skill and fluency, one should live among people who speak a language well and speak it constantly. No translation is necessary. One learns each language in terms of its own grammar, vocabulary, and idioms by speaking it.

So it is with the inverted image of indirect ophthalmoscopy. Most of us come to the indirect technique after mastering the direct one. Some of us have achieved great facility and experience with direct ophthalmoscopy and a few have even acquired great reputation for this skill. It is natural to attempt to translate into familiar erect-image terms the unfamiliar image of indirect ophthalmoscopy. Not until we break away absolutely from direct ophthalmoscopic concepts is it possible to learn orientation with indirect ophthalmoscopy. This means frustration during the trying period when the new "vocabulary" and "idioms" are being acquired.

If we can agree to avoid comparisons between the direct and indirect fundus images, what then is the method to learn orientation with the unfamiliar inverted image?

Drawing of the Fundus Just as constant practice of a foreign language is the key to incorporating it into one's unconscious thought processes, so drawing of the fundus is the key technique to mastery of the inverted image. In our experience teaching indirect ophthalmoscopy, we have never seen anyone master indirect ophthalmoscopy in any expert sense who did not draw the fundus. Most people who think they can see well with the indirect technique are chagrined to find how much they are not seeing when they are confronted by a drawing of that fundus. Most of us are filled with numerous resistances and rationalizations for not attempting to draw. One hears such things as "I cannot draw," "I am not an artist," or "I see it, why do I have to draw it?" The simple fact is that if you cannot draw a fundus lesion, you do not really see it. If the author is emphatic on this point, it is only because his own initial resistance to drawing was so strong and so unfounded. It is not necessary to be artistic in any sense to make useful fundus sketches. The important thing is not the sketch itself but the process of making it. In some way that is not obvious, the attempt to put down on paper what one is seeing forces us to perceive detail we cannot make out in any other way. The problem of orientation in the fundus will be solved by learning to accurately draw the image that we see in the condensing lens.

We shall approach the problem of making the fundus drawing in a purely mechanical manner. No attempt will be made to invert the fundus image before we put it down on paper. Rather, we will attempt to accurately reproduce the picture that we see in the condensing lens exactly as it appears. It will be remembered that the fundus image in the condensing lens is completely inverted; that is, the image is upside down and also backwards as regards right and left (Figure 22). We will therefore take the drawing chart upon which we will represent the patient's fundus and invert that on the patient's chest. Figure 23 shows the relationship of the fundus chart to the patient's eye. It will be seen that the 6-o'clock position on the chart faces up toward the pa-

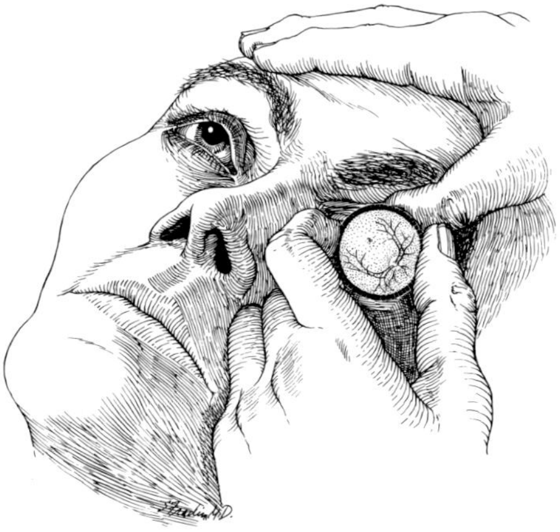

Figure 22 *Left eye is being examined. Image is condensing lens of disc, and macula is inverted. In drawing this image, it should be copied just as seen on inverted drawing chart. Inverted image is drawn on inverted chart, thus preserving normal relationships.*

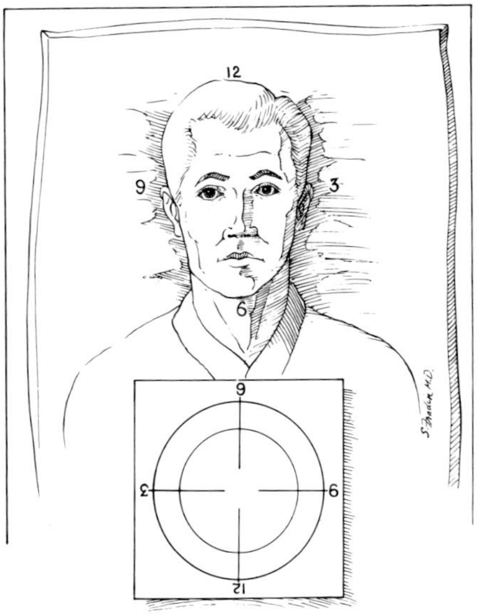

Figure 23 *Chart is placed, inverted, on supine patient's chest. It can be seen that 12-o'clock position on chart corresponds to 6-o'clock position on patient's eye. Likewise, 6-o'clock position on chart corresponds to 12-o'clock position on patient's eye. However, when fundus is viewed through condensing lens, inverted image in lens will exactly correspond to orientation of chart. Information in lens image can be directly drawn on inverted chart.*

tient's head. The 9-o'clock and 3-o'clock meridians on the fundus chart are also inversely related to 9 o'clock and 3 o'clock in the patient's eye. A moment's thought will convince the student that the drawing paper is now inverted regarding the patient's fundus. Since the image in the lens is also inverted regarding the fundus, the image in the lens now corresponds exactly to the drawing chart. Therefore, if we merely transpose directly what we see in the lens to the drawing paper, all relationships will be correctly obtained. No attempt should be made to think in terms such as superior, inferior, or temporal or nasal when performing this operation initially. These concepts become confusing when dealing with an inverted image. In other words, the observer should think only in terms of posterior in the fundus and anterior in the fundus, or central and peripheral. No matter on what side of the patient's eye the observer stands, whatever appears closest to the observer in the condensing lens (down in the lens) is peripheral in the fundus compared with a fundus object that is farther away from the observer in the condensing lens (up in the lens). As the observer moves around the fundus, he should constantly analyze the fundus image in the lens in terms of peripheral and central and disregard completely for the time being the meridian that he is observing. The previously described exercise of observing the disc and following a vessel out to the equator, with the proper body and hand coordination, will serve to clarify how peripheral parts of the fundus come into view from the proximal part of the lens (which is

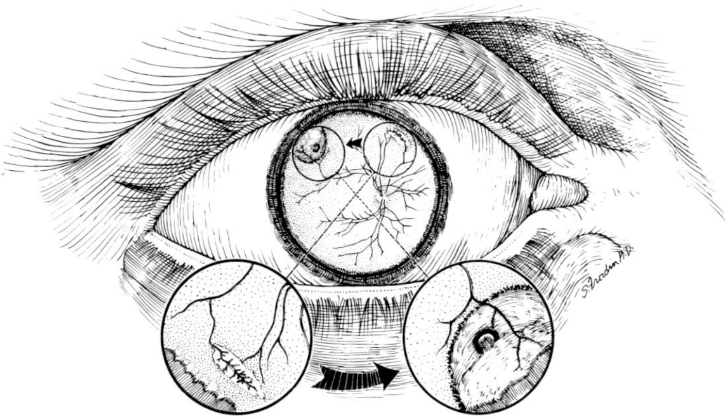

Figure 24 *Fundus of right eye is shown. Fundus is seen directly as if cornea was removed, and lesions are shown as they actually are in fundus. We can see two fields of interest: localized retinal detachment with demarcation line and horseshoe tear at 11-o'clock position, and patch of lattice degeneration of retina at 1-o'clock position. Beneath eye we see two fields as seen in condensing lens of indirect ophthalmoscope. It should be noted that in each case we see field of view inverted as if we were standing on ora serrata looking back toward posterior pole. Actually, we are observing each of these lesions from opposite position, or 180° away. As we move in fundus from view of 11-o'clock lesion, toward 1-o'clock field, 12-o'clock and then 1-o'clock areas come into view from left side of condensing lens.*

down). As one sweeps back toward the disc from the equator, the more posterior parts of the fundus come back into view from the superior part of the lens.

Position Between Observer and Lesion Being Examined One should attempt, when drawing a specific object in the fundus on the fundus chart, to stand 180° away from the lesion being observed. This will serve to simplify the observer's understanding of the proper meridian along which to draw the lesion on the chart. A few minutes' consideration of this problem will serve to clarify it. If we imagine a lesion at the 11-o'clock position in the patient's fundus, we should stand inferiorly and look superiorly toward that lesion (Figure 24). One will observe in the lens that the disc appears in the upper part of the condensing lens and the lesion appears below it, and this is as it should be, since more peripheral objects appear down in the lens as previously stated. If we then glance down at the drawing chart, we will see that we

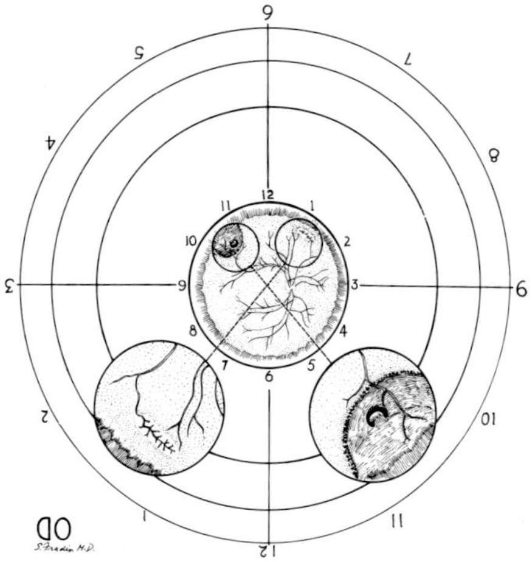

Figure 25 *Large circle represents inverted fundus chart upon which we will draw. Smaller central circle is direct view of eye from previous figure. Numbers around smaller circle show true meridians in that fundus. Drawings in two lower circles represent fields at 11-o'clock and 1-o'clock positions, respectively, as seen in condensing lens. These views in condensing lens should be drawn directly on chart from position at which examiner stands to see field. Therefore, field seen at 1-o'clock position, since it is observed while standing at 7-o'clock position with respect to patient, is drawn at 7-o'clock position on inverted chart as shown. Note that inverted meridians on drawing chart are disregarded at first. However, if one now considers true meridians, it will be noted that if chart is turned right side up field drawn will be in precisely correct place.*

are standing near the meridian we are observing, that is, the 11-o'clock meridian (Figure 25). If we move over and look at an object at the 12-o'clock position in the fundus, we will see that we are standing close to the 12-o'clock meridian on the fundus drawing. If we observe a lesion at the 3-o'clock position, we will be standing at the 9-o'clock meridian in reference to the patient's eye, but we will be standing at the 3-o'clock meridian on the fundus chart. From this fact we can derive an important guide rule in placing objects that we see in the condensing lens on the fundus chart. This rule is that we should draw the image that we see in the lens as we observe it from 180° away, on that part of the fundus chart which is closest to us (see Figures 24, 25). We should begin by drawing an initial landmark, which could be a vessel or a specific spot; once we have drawn one landmark, it is easy to relate subsequent fundus landmarks to the original one. In the example being considered of a lesion at the 11-o'clock position, reasonably close to the disc, we would transpose the image to the fundus drawing exactly as seen. The disc is already marked on the fundus chart and we therefore would place the lesion below it just as we see it in the lens. If another lesion is present at the 1-o'clock position in the fundus, it will come into view from the left-hand side of the condensing lens and will be drawn to the left of the original lesion on the fundus drawing. It will be seen that this will place it at the correct 1-o'clock meridian on the chart. Similarly, a lesion at the 9-o'clock position will come into view from the right-hand side of the lens and it will be drawn on the fundus drawing to the right of the previous two lesions. This also will be correctly placed on the fundus drawing at the 9-o'clock meridian. The vessels running toward these lesions should be drawn exactly as they appear in the lens. If the drawing is now picked up and reinverted, it will be seen that a drawing has been made that is exactly the same as if it had been drawn by direct ophthalmoscopy. We have drawn an inverted drawing of an inverted image. By repeating this process over and over again, one develops a subconscious familiarity with relationships of fundus landmarks in the condensing lens (Figures 26, 27). It becomes easier and easier to accurately reproduce what one sees in the condensing lens, and gradually the problem of the inverted image seems less important. When enough drawings have been made, and for most observers this is about 25 fundus drawings, the problem of orientation completely disappears and one is no longer troubled by the inverted image at all.

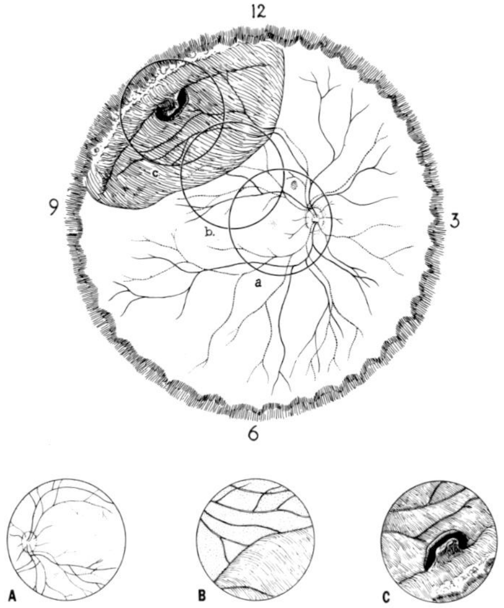

Figure 26 *In large figure we note direct view of right fundus which includes superotemporal retinal detachment. Small circles within larger one represent three fields to be studied with indirect ophthalmoscope. These fields are labeled A, B, and C. Three circles below large figure show appearance in condensing lens of respective fundus fields with image inverted.*

Do We Actually See the Specific Area of the Fundus We Are Observing or the Area Opposite to It? Some ophthalmologists are confused as to what we are actually seeing when we look in a specific direction in the fundus. The question is often, "If I look up and temporal in the patient's eye, since the image is inverted, do I see the lower nasal part of the fundus?" The answer is "absolutely not." You always see that area which you are looking at, whether using a direct or

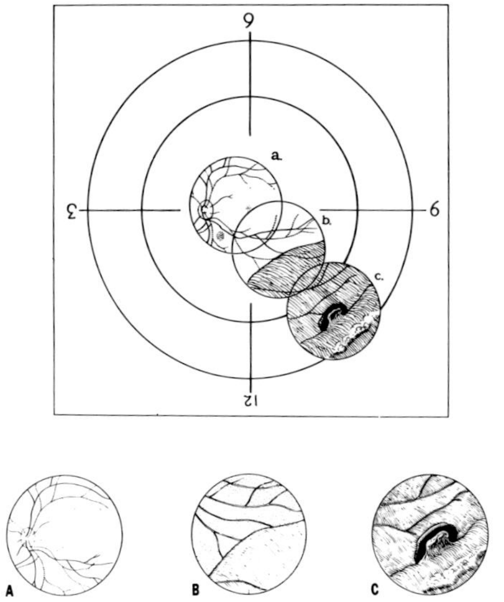

Figure 27 *Three circles below large figure (A, B, C) show condensing lens fields of view as noted in previous figure. In large figure, it should be noted that in view C, ora serrata is found in lower part of lens, since it is most peripheral, and in view A, disc is found in upper part of lens, since it is most posterior. It can be seen that in view B, most posterior edge of detachment comes in view from upper part of lens. These fields are drawn on inverted fundus chart as indicated.*

indirect ophthalmoscope. However, whatever field you see in the condensing lens will be inverted.

Another way of considering this matter is as follows:

We see whichever meridian of the fundus we look at as if we were standing on the ora serrata at that meridian, looking toward the posterior pole of the eye. Thus, if we look toward the 12-o'clock part of the fundus, we see the 12-o'clock region as if we were standing on the ora serrata at the 12-o'clock position.

Fundus Charts Fundus drawings should be made on standard fundus charts, which can be obtained from many sources. These charts should be large enough so that adequate detail can be reproduced. They should show all the meridians numbered by the clock. The equator and the ora serrata line should be present, as well as a line indicating the extreme limit of view with depression on the ciliary body. Such a chart is reproduced in Figures 28 and 29. Colored pencils are useful in giving a clear, concise reproduction of fundus pathology. It is now ordinarily possible to represent with artistic fidelity the fundi we are examining. Most retinal clinics in the United States have agreed upon a standard color code, which is reproduced in Figure 30. It is convenient to use the correct color according to the code. This method will result in drawings that have meaning to other people familiar with the code and serve as a good record for the observer to measure his progress in funduscopy. The drawings also have obvious clinical importance as a record of the patient's fundus.

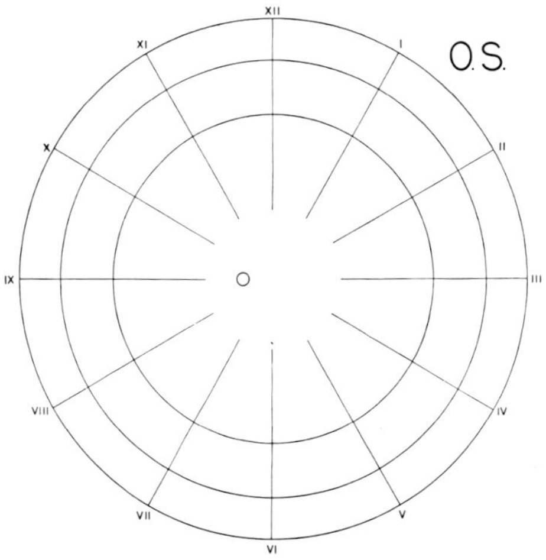

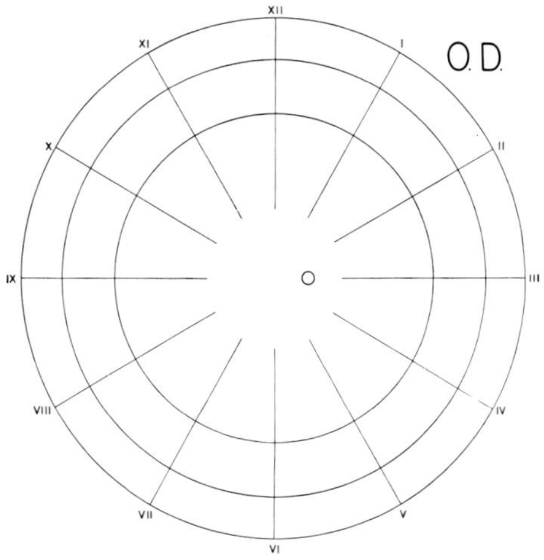

Figure 28 *Chart contains three concentric circles. Inner circle represents equator, middle circle represents ora serrata, and outer circle represents region of ciliary processes. Band between middle and outer circles is pars plana of ciliary body. Small circle in center of chart represents disc.*

Figure 29 *(Top right) Fundus drawing chart for right eye.*

Figure 30 *(Right) Standard key to colors in fundus sketch. [The currently recommended color code is discussed in Section 3-9; see also Figure 3-2 and Table 3-2.]*

Blue	Detached retina
	Retinal veins
Red	Attached retina
	Retinal arteries
	Hemorrhage in retina
Red Lined With Blue	Retinal breaks
Black	Retinal pigmentation
	Choroidal pigmentation when seen through attached retina
Brown	Choroidal pigmentation seen through detached retina
Green	Opacities in media, including vitreous hemorrhage
Yellow	Chorioretinal exudation
	Macular edema

SCLERAL DEPRESSION

Until now we have concerned ourselves with studying and drawing only that part of the fundus which lies posterior to the equator. Only when the student has mastered the technique of drawing this part of the fundus is he ready to attempt scleral depression. This statement cannot be overemphasized. If the student has not mastered the problems of moving the hand–head axis, he cannot possibly line up an additional element, the depressor, on the axis (see Figure 19). Premature attempts at scleral depression usually result in the observer being frustrated in his attempt to see the mound of the depressor in the fundus because of poor alignment. The novice then usually presses more vigorously, resulting in patient pain and lack of cooperation.

Purposes of Scleral Depression

The technique of scleral depression has two main functions. The first is to make visible that part of the fundus which lies anterior to the equator. This region is ordinarily not visible at all without the use of scleral depression. A second and perhaps even more important function is to enable the observer to palpate the retina and to examine critically the equatorial region of the fundus, which is frequently visible without the use of scleral depression but which can only be critically evaluated with scleral depression. The anatomy and pathologic anatomy of the far retinal periphery is, of course, unfamiliar to an individual who has not previously seen it. There is a wide variation in the appearance of the region of the ora serrata in eyes of various types. We must examine large numbers of fundus peripheries before we may truly appreciate the variations within normal eyes, as well as various types of pathology.

Holding the Instrument for Scleral Depression

The instrument which is best suited for use as a scleral depressor consists of a small, curved shaft with a flattened knob-like tip mounted on a thimble. This instrument is demonstrated in Figure 31. The instrument can be grasped in several ways. It can be held between the thumb and index finger, or it can be placed upon the index or middle finger as shown in Figure 31. Each method of holding the depressor has certain advantages and can be used at different times to afford facility.

Examining the Ora Serrata

In attempting scleral depression for the first time, it is well to try to see a part of the ora serrata region that is (1) clearly identifiable and (2) more easily seen than other areas of the ora.

The typical ora teeth and bays that one commonly visualizes when thinking of the ora serrata are really only typical of the nasal ora. In this region, the nasal ora appears as in Figure 32B. The characteristic teeth and bays are seen, and the characteristic distribution of pigment in the pars plana in this region can also be noted. The temporal ora serrata (Figure 32A) does not have noticeable ora teeth and bays, and the pigment band on the pars plana is somewhat thicker and more pronounced. Cystoid degeneration is usually more prominent than on the nasal side. The demarcation between retina and ciliary epithelium is less clearly marked temporally than it is nasally, and it is much easier for the inexperienced observer to recognize and appreciate the ora on the nasal side. Furthermore, the absence of an overhanging orbital margin superonasally and nasally makes it easier for the scleral depressor to be applied here than on the temporal side. We therefore recommend that initial attempts at scleral depression be made superonasally.

For this purpose, the patient is positioned exactly as described previously for examination of the superior part of the fundus (see Figure 15). The scleral depressor should be grasped between the thumb and the index finger, and the patient should be asked to look down. The depressor should be applied to the superior lid, without pressure, at the tarsal margin (Figure 33). The patient then should be asked to look up and, as the superior lid retracts, the depressor should be slid posteriorly, parallel to the surface of the globe (Figure 34).

The depressor now lies against the globe held by the thumb and forefinger, and no pressure is being applied to the globe. The light from the ophthalmoscope is now projected onto the fundus superonasally, the condensing lens is interposed, and the fundus at the equator is brought into view. The depressor should now be

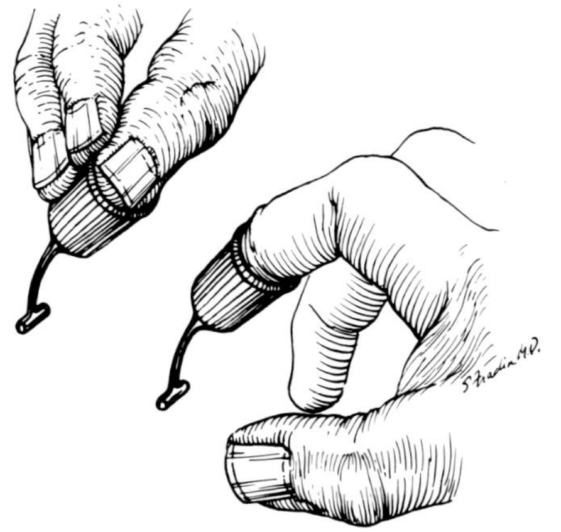

A

B

Figure 31 *Two most satisfactory techniques for manipulating scleral depressor are shown. (A) Shows method that is easier to learn for most people because it closely resembles way pencil or ophthalmic surgical instrument is held. (B) This method is better for certain situations, such as when third finger is needed to hold patient's lid.*

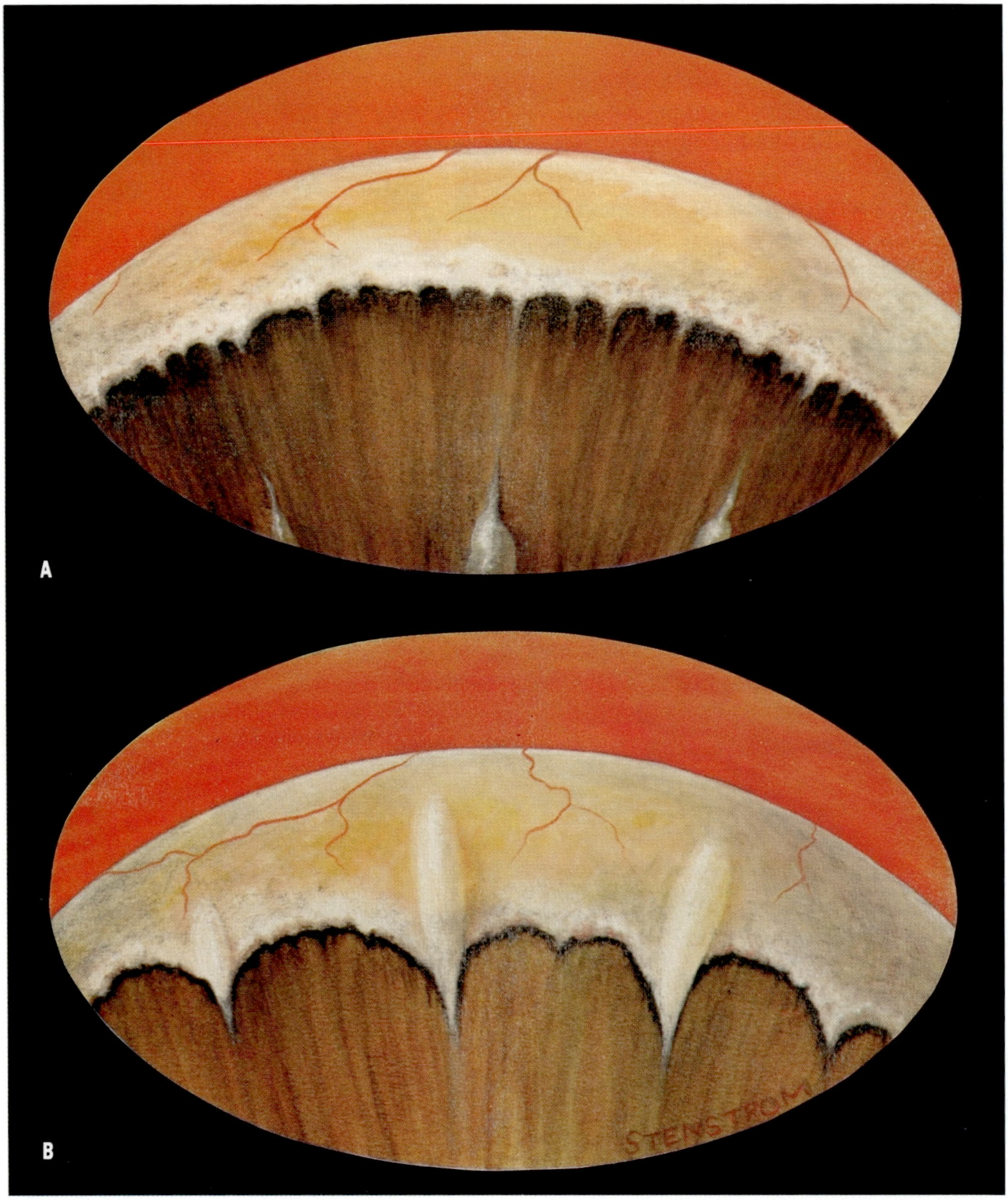

Figure 32 *(A) Temporal ora serrata. (B) Nasal ora serrata.*

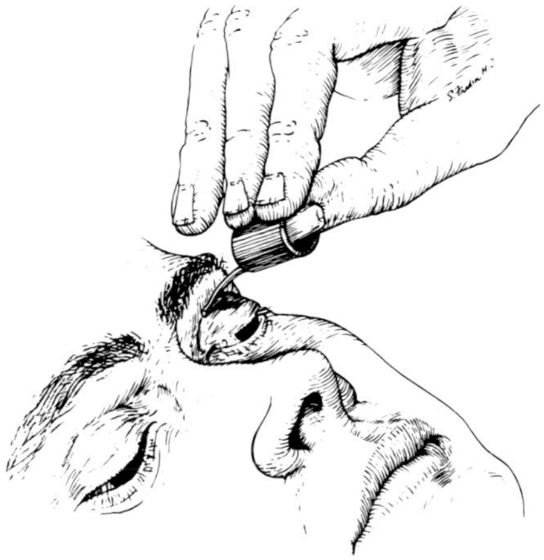

Figure 33 *Shows depressor being applied to patient's eye, with patient looking down. When patient looks up and depressor is introduced, examiner will be in position to see superonasal periphery.*

Figure 34 *(A) Depressor being applied to upper lid at tarsal margin while patient looks down. Shaft of instrument is parallel to surface of globe. No pressure is being applied to eye at this time. (B) Patient has been asked to look up, and depressor has been advanced into orbit alongside globe. Shaft of instrument is still parallel to surface of globe, and no pressure is as yet being applied to eye. (C) Shows tip of instrument being depressed gently, producing mound in fundus. Note that at all stages depressor is approximately parallel to globe and is inserted well back in orbit so that initial depression occurs at equator. Parallel position minimizes danger of excessive pressure, and posterior position avoids pressure on limbus; errors of technique on both of these phases of examination cause pain.*

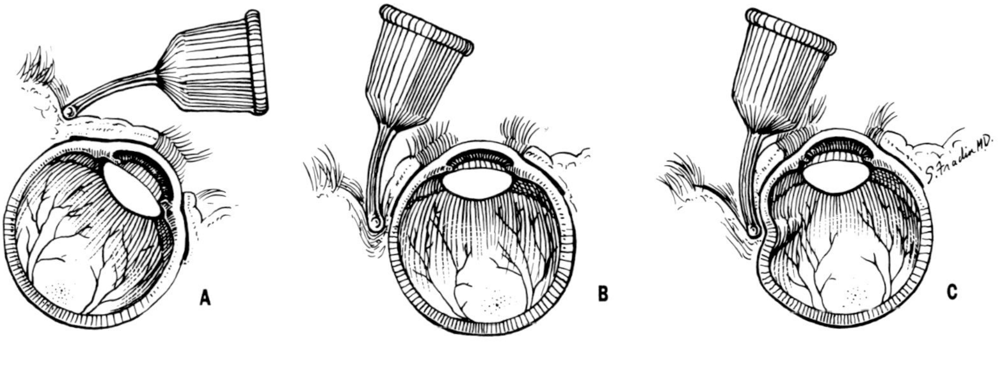

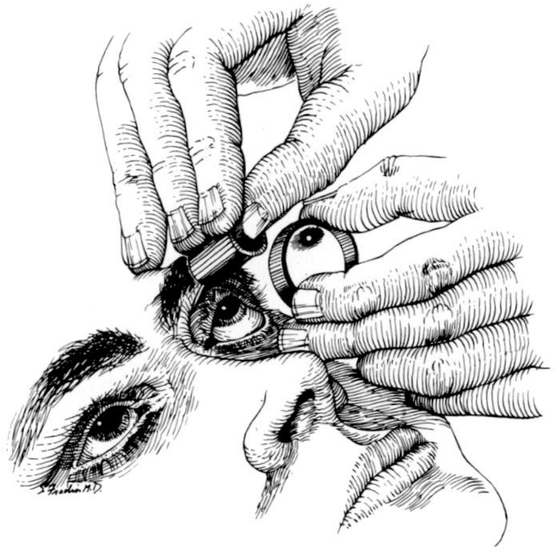

Figure 35 *Scleral depressor and condensing lens in position to examine superonasal fundus. Note use of fourth finger of examiner's right hand in steadying depressor in same way that third, fourth, and fifth fingers of left hand steady lens.*

gently pressed against the globe at the equatorial region and, if it is applied in the correct meridian, a grayish mound comes into view from the inferior part of the lens. This is to be expected, since our depression is anterior and we will always see it as a bulge in the fundus appearing in the lower part of the condensing lens. A small adjustment in the lens should now bring into clear focus the image of this depressed and indented part of the fundus. The patient should be asked to look superonasally, and the depressor should be slid anteriorly and slowly under direct visual control. The ora serrata should slide into view in the inferior part of the lens (Figure 35; see also Figure 32B).

The amount of pressure necessary to see the fundus with the depressor will vary slightly with the intraocular pressure of the eye being examined. However, in general, the amount of pressure is about the same as that used when estimating intraocular pressure by taction. Most beginners use too much pressure; in no case should the pressure be so great that the patient is uncomfortable. A person who is skilled with this technique can examine even young children without causing them any discomfort.

Once the image of the indented part of the fundus is in view, farther parts of the fundus are brought into view by direct visual control. One moves the depressor, the lens, and the observer's head in a coordinated manner to move from one part of the retinal periphery to another. It is important to emphasize that the observer's eye, the eyepiece of the ophthalmoscope, the condensing lens, the patient's pupil, the object being studied in the fundus, and the scleral depressor all must lie on a straight line as indicated in Figure 19. The depressor should be applied in a direction as parallel to this axis as possible. It is not satisfactory to depress with the instrument at a great angle to this viewing axis.

In the majority of instances, scleral depression should be performed through the lids (Figure 36). Even the 9-o'clock and 3-o'clock meridians can be examined in most patients by careful application of the depressor on the superior lids. If the lid is lax, it can be dragged down slightly with the depressor to enable these meridians to be examined (see Figures 36B,C). In some cases, however, it may be necessary to examine the 9-o'clock and 3-o'clock meridians by direct application of the scleral depressor to the bulbar conjunctiva (Figure 37). If this is necessary, it will be observed that even less pressure is necessary to see the fundus than if one applies the pressure through the lids. It is generally not necessary to use a local anesthetic when applying the depressor on the bulbar conjunctiva. It is never necessary to use a topical anesthetic when applying the depressor to the lids. If an occasional patient cannot tolerate the scleral depressor applied directly to the conjunctiva at the 9-o'clock and 3-o'clock positions, a drop or two of a suitable topical anesthetic will enable this maneuver to be performed. The amount of pressure necessary to see the superior periphery is somewhat less than that necessary to see the inferior periphery due to the somewhat greater thickness of the inferior lid.

In examining the ora serrata region, it is usually necessary to have the patient

A

B

C

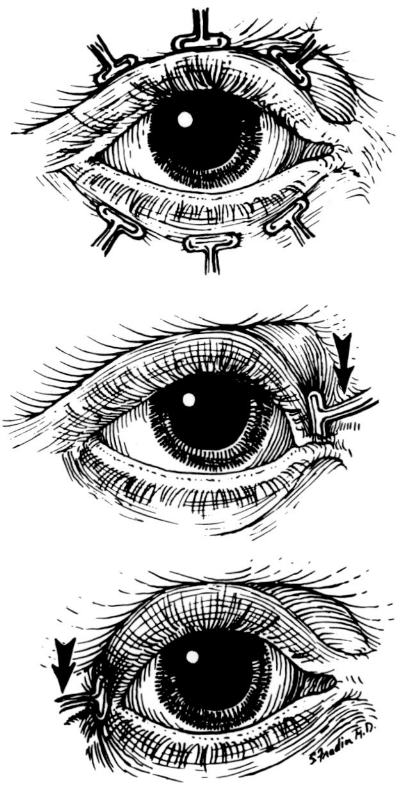

Figure 36 *(A) Shows the approximately six positions of depressor on lids, sufficient to provide view of entire periphery with exception of 9- and 3-o'clock positions. (B) Shows how, in most patients, it is possible to drag upper lid down enough to visualize nasal horizontal meridian. (C) Shows how it is usually possible to drag upper lid down enough to examine temporal horizontal meridian.*

Figure 37 *In cases where lids are tight, or patient is squeezer, it may be necessary to apply depressor directly to globe in order to examine the 9- and 3-o'clock meridians. Technique is as follows: With patient looking straight ahead, depressor is introduced into lateral or nasal fornix parallel to globe. Patient is then asked to look to right or left, as case may be, and depressor follows eye back, just as in case of examining superior fundus. As long as depressor does not touch cornea, this is painless procedure. Topical anesthesia is not usually needed.*

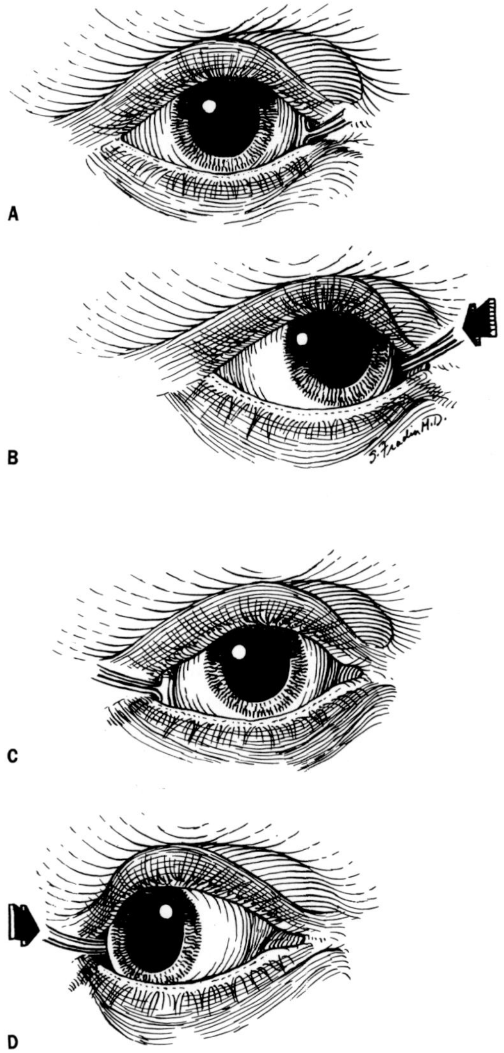

look toward the meridian one wishes to examine. However, it is important to emphasize the necessity for the observer to move his own body freely in examining the retinal periphery. In examining the ora serrata, it is usually necessary to tilt the condensing lens somewhat forward into a plane more nearly parallel to the iris. It is also sometimes necessary to tilt the light of the ophthalmoscope somewhat higher and tilt the mirror or eyepiece by adjusting the control screw of the mirror. One soon learns to make these adjustments without thinking. When applying pressure with the depressor, it is important to apply such pressure with the depressor parallel to the globe. Pressure should be applied as shown in Figure 34.

Another frequent error the beginner makes is to apply his depressor too far anteriorly; this causes considerable discomfort to the patient and, of course, will not permit visualization of the retina.

Having now achieved a view of the ora serrata, we must practice the manipulation necessary to control the movement of the fundus mound by direct visual control while looking in the condensing lens. When we achieve some facility in moving from one place to another, we are then able to appreciate the real value of scleral depression.

It must be emphasized that scleral depression is a dynamic and not a static technique. Significant help in interpreting fundus pathology is obtained by changes in the fundus produced by movements of the scleral depressor. The experienced observer is constantly moving the depressor with fine massaging movements anterior, posterior, and also sideways. These slight movements enable the observer to move lesions in the fundus and to examine them from many directions rapidly. This technique is sometimes referred to as "rolling" a lesion. It is this dynamic aspect of scleral depression that enables one to pick up lesions in the fundus that are invisible without scleral depression.

The use of depression allows us to detect and differentiate raised lesions from depressed lesions in the fundus and to determine the difference between a hemorrhage and a retinal break. It also enables us to see a retinal break that is invisible until the depressor is applied under it. Figure 38 shows how the movement of the depressor produces changes in the fundus mound, which in turn change the view one gets of a fundus lesion. Figure 38A shows the appearance of the lesion without the use of the scleral depressor. Figure 38B shows the appearance of the lesion with the scleral depressor in place, with the apex of the mound at approximately the equator. Well down on the anterior slope of the mound, one sees a round red lesion that is difficult to identify. After the depressor is slid anteriorly (Figure 38C), the nondescript red spot is brought up to the crest of the mound. At this point, it is seen to be a break in the retina (see Figure 38C). The depression has blanched the margins of the retinal break and increased the contrast between the edges of the break and the subjacent choroid.

Figure 38 *(A) Appearance of retinal lesion without use of scleral depression. (B) Shows view of fundus in condensing lens, with scleral depressor in place. Crest of mound thus produced is posterior to round red lesion seen on mound. Round gray disc floats in vitreous over mound in fundus and casts shadow on retina. Exact nature of red lesion cannot be made out in this view. It could be either hemorrhage in retina or retinal break. (C) Shows change in appearance which occurs when depressor is moved anterior enough to position lesion precisely on crest of mound. In this view, sharp edge of lesion identifies it as retinal break. Small gray disc in vitreous is now identifiable as operculum—piece of retina torn out of break by vitreous traction. If red lesion in this example were cyst rather than tear, it would appear on mound as little lump. If it were merely flat hemorrhage, no change in surface contour would be detected.*

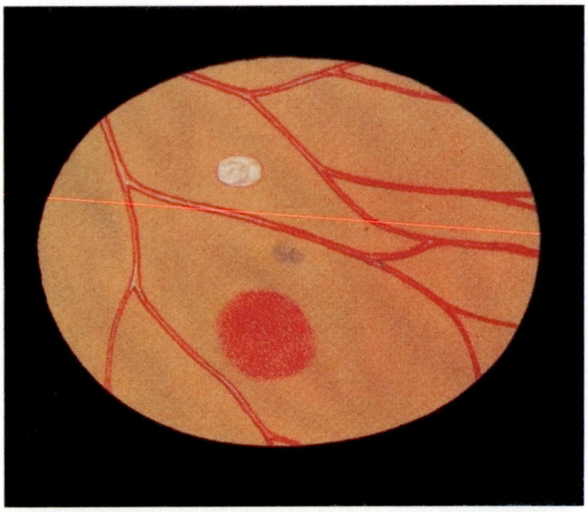

A

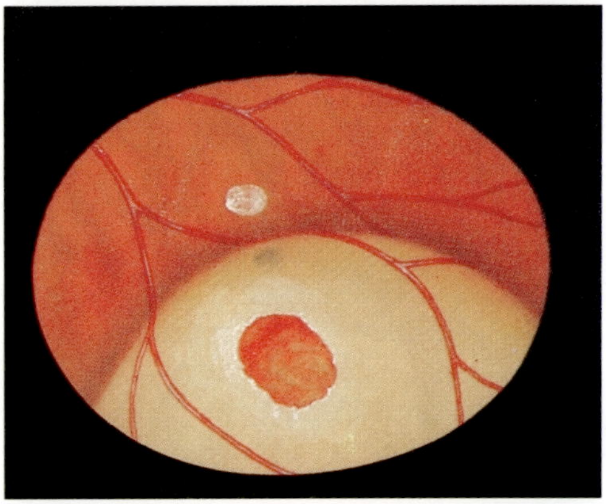

B

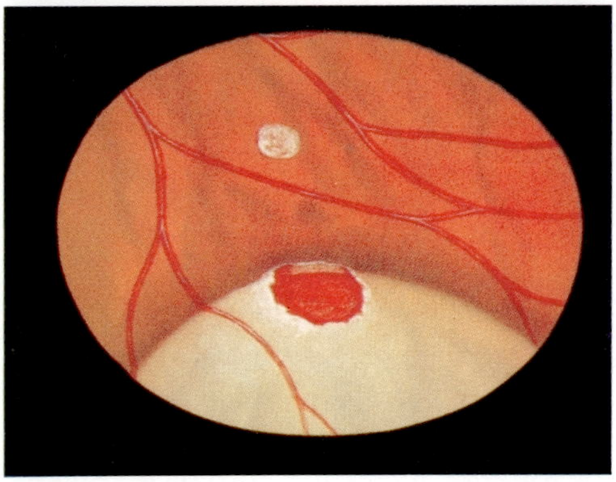

C

It must be emphasized that it is the fine movements of the depressor that bring out details of fundus lesions. With this technique, it should be possible, in an eye whose pupil dilates normally, to examine the ora serrata for 360° and the posterior one third of the pars plana ciliaris. In hypotonic eyes and in aphakic eyes, it is generally possible to examine somewhat more of the ciliary body than the posterior one third.

Details in Fundus Drawing

The question frequently arises as to how much detail the student should include in his drawing of the fundus. The answer is that the more effort expended in drawing detail, the greater the reward in terms of development of a reflex skill. The student should at least draw all veins in great detail, paying great attention to small changes in the vessel directions, and to the accurate reproduction of branch relationships. Any distinctive pigmented areas or patterned areas should be accurately reproduced. The attempt to accurately copy details of form in fundus lesions is particularly rewarding. If a detachment of the retina is present, it is important to reproduce accurately the shape of a dominant retinal fold system, the position and shape of the retinal breaks, and their relationships to the retinal vessels and other fixed landmarks.

In order to be certain that no area of the fundus escapes examination, a system of examination is essential. It is not important what system is chosen, but it is necessary to choose a specific system and adhere to it. Otherwise, one is likely to fail to see lesions of considerable size and importance. We can start by drawing the fundus posterior to the equator, hour by hour on the dial. If we draw every retinal vein out to the equator, this method should assure careful coverage of this area. The area between the equator and the ora serrata is then examined separately by going around the eye, hour by hour with the scleral depressor, placing lesions on the chart in careful relationship to vessels previously drawn.

If a retinal detachment is present, it is usually best to chart out the dominant features of the detachment, whatever they may be. Frequently, the balloons have a characteristic shape and can be plotted as a scaffold upon which to place the vessels and the retinal breaks. If fixed folds dominate the picture, they often can be used as a skeleton. In any case, the dominant topographic features should be laid down as a framework and then the fundus examined in detail out to the equator. The area between the equator and the ora serrata region is approached as previously described. Particular attention must be given to the 9-o'clock and 3-o'clock meridians, since lesions at or anterior to the equator in these meridians are easy to overlook due to the technical difficulty of applying the scleral depressor here.

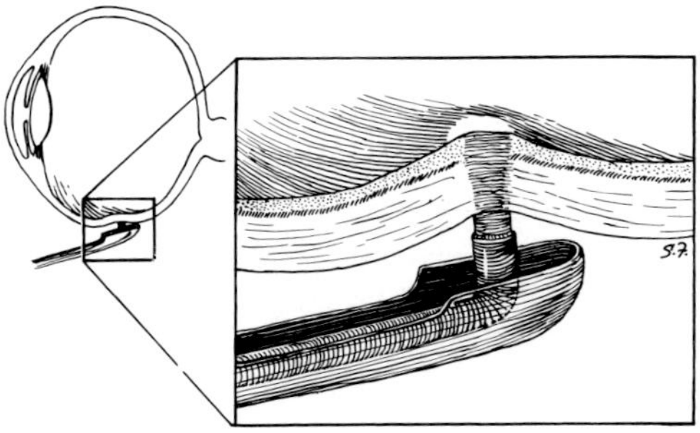

Figure 39 *Arruga retractor is slipped in place between eye and wall of orbit. This maintains dry working area. Flat, nonpenetrating surface electrode is used as scleral depressor to produce mound in fundus (see Figure 40B). When crest of mound is precisely where desired (see Figure 40B), current is turned on, and scleral burn and usually retina mark (see Figures 40B,C) will result. Scleral mark is precise guide on sclera to position in fundus of retinal mark. In order to perform this maneuver, considerable facility with scleral depression must be acquired in dark room.*

Technique in the Operating Room

Even after considerable skill has been acquired in the aforementioned methods, performing these maneuvers in the operating room will be a cause of new frustrations.

The position of the patient on the operating table may not be entirely satisfactory. The drapes hinder access to the eye to some extent. The examiner's gown and gloves will be a handicap. The nurse may have instilled medications on the eye that may cause slight corneal epithelial edema, unless the surgeon has warned her previously not to do so.

All of these minor hazards may add up to a major difficulty in seeing the fundus at the most critical time.

It is important to adjust the table height to your satisfaction. Usually it is too high for ophthalmoscopy if left at the height that is comfortable for surgery. No drops except dilating medication should be placed in the eye.

Scleral depression in the operating room is best performed by using a cotton-tipped applicator stick, which is left dry or almost dry. The applicator stick is used to position the eye and simultaneously depress the sclera. When a localizing diathermy mark is desired on the sclera, the fundus lesion is first localized with the cotton stick. Then an Arruga plastic retractor is introduced by an assistant into the orbit so as to straddle the stick. The cotton stick is then removed, without moving the eye. A flat diathermy elec-

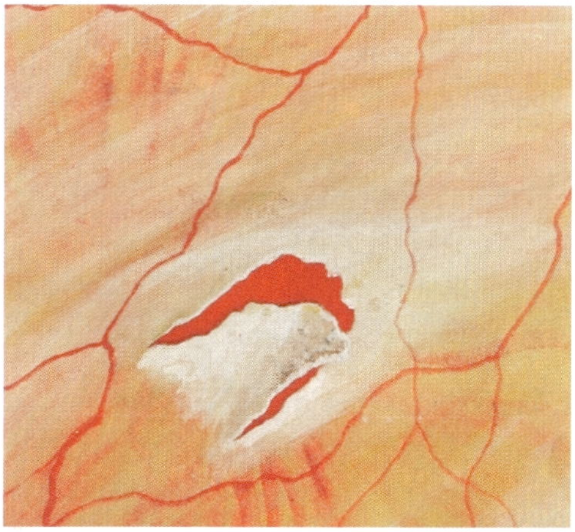

A

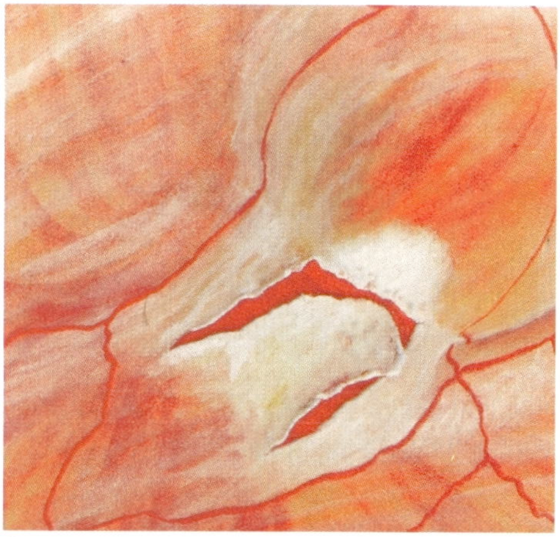

B

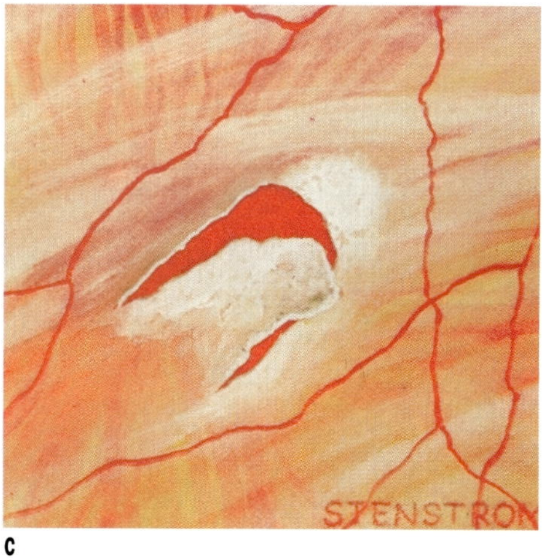

C

Figure 40 *Use of diathermy electrode to localize fundus lesions in operating room.*

trode is then introduced under ophthalmoscopic control, and scleral depression is performed with it (Figure 39) until the mound in the fundus caused by the electrode is positioned to the examiner's satisfaction (Figure 40B). The current is then turned on and a burn on the sclera results. If the retina was not too highly detached, a retinal burn will also result, corresponding exactly to the scleral burn (Figure 40C). Even if the retinal burn is not seen, if the fundus mound produced by the electrode was seen to be in the right position (see Figure 40C), the scleral mark is an accurate indication of the position of the retinal lesion (see Figure 39).

The same procedure can be used to mark the scleral site for the removal of an intraocular foreign body, or to place perforating diathermy in a retinoblastoma.

CME Accreditation

The American Academy of Ophthalmology is accredited by the Accreditation Council for Continuing Medical Education to sponsor continuing medical education for physicians.

CME credit hours in Category 1 of the Physician's Recognition Award of the American Medical Association may be earned for completing the study of any monograph in the Ophthalmology Monographs series. The Academy designates the number of credit hours for each monograph based on the scope and complexity of the material covered.

CME Credit Report Form

The Academy designates Ophthalmology Monograph 1, *Retinal Detachment: Principles and Practice*, Second Edition, for up to 25 credit hours. To claim credit, complete the answer sheet for the self-study examination and sign the statement below.

I hereby certify that I have spent _____ (up to 25) hours of study on this monograph and that I have completed the self-study examination.

Signature ______________________ Date ____________

Send the completed answer sheet and signed statement to:

American Academy of Ophthalmology
P.O. Box 7424
San Francisco, CA 94120-7424
ATTN: Clinical Education Division

The Academy upon request will send you a transcript of the credit claimed on this form. Check the box below if you wish credit verification now.

☐ Please send credit verification now.

PLEASE PRINT

Last Name ______________________ First Name ______________________ MI ____

Mailing Address ______________________

City ______________________

State ______________________ ZIP Code ____________

Telephone ______________________ ID Number* ____________

*Your ID Number is located following your name on most Academy mailing labels, in your membership directory, and on your monthly statement of account.

OPHTHALMOLOGY MONOGRAPH 1, Second Edition

Retinal Detachment: Principles and Practice

Circle the letter of the response option that you regard as the "best" answer to the question.

Question	Answer				
1	a	b	c	d	e
2	a	b	c	d	e
3	a	b	c	d	e
4	a	b	c	d	e
5	a	b	c	d	e
6	a	b	c	d	e
7	a	b	c	d	e
8	a	b	c	d	e
9	a	b	c	d	e
10	a	b	c	d	e
11	a	b	c	d	e
12	a	b	c	d	e
13	a	b	c	d	e
14	a	b	c	d	e
15	a	b	c	d	e
16	a	b	c	d	e
17	a	b	c	d	e
18	a	b	c	d	e
19	a	b	c	d	e
20	a	b	c	d	e

SELF-STUDY EXAMINATION

The self-study examination provided for each book in the Ophthalmology Monographs series is intended for use after completion of the monograph. The examination for *Retinal Detachment: Principles and Practice*, Second Edition, consists of 20 multiple-choice questions followed by the answers to the questions and a discussion of each answer. The Academy recommends that you not consult the answers until you have completed the entire examination.

Questions

The questions are constructed so that there is one "best" answer for each. Despite the attempt to avoid ambiguous selections, disagreement may occur about which selection constitutes the optimal answer. After reading a question, record your initial impression on the answer sheet (facing page).

Answers and Discussions

The "best" answer to each question is provided after the examination. The discussion that accompanies the answer is intended to help you confirm that the reasoning you used in determining the most appropriate answer was correct. If you missed a question, the discussion may help you decide whether your "error" was due to poor wording of the question or to your misinterpretation. If, instead, you missed the question because of miscalculation or failure to recall relevant information, the discussion may help fix the principle in your memory.

QUESTIONS

1. All of the following conditions commonly affect visual acuity after successful surgery for retinal detachment *except*

a. macular pucker

b. cystoid macular edema

c. derangement of the retinal pigment epithelium

d. pigment "fallout" from cryotherapy

e. subretinal hemorrhage

2. The problem most feared following surgery for retinal detachment is

a. subretinal hemorrhage

b. preretinal membrane formation

c. diplopia

d. myopic refractive error

e. cataract formation

3. Common complications of scleral buckling include all of the following *except*

a. astigmatism

b. myopia

c. diplopia

d. hyperopia

e. ptosis

4. The preoperative factor most important in predicting postoperative visual acuity after successful retinal reattachment surgery is

a. macular involvement

b. proliferative vitreoretinopathy

c. pseudophakia

d. preoperative visual acuity

e. duration of retinal detachment

5. Most recurrent retinal detachments can be successfully repaired with multiple procedures unless the cause of the redetachment is due to

a. new retinal breaks

b. severe epiretinal membrane formation

c. "inadequate" scleral buckles

d. "inadequate" chorioretinal adhesions

e. choroidal detachments

6. After successful reattachment surgery for retinal detachment with preoperative macular involvement, the average patient can expect that visual acuity will return to approximately

a. 20/30

b. 20/50

c. 20/70

d. 20/200

e. 20/400

7. Over the past 45 years, which of the following has been most responsible for improved anatomic results in surgery for retinal detachment?

a. the binocular indirect ophthalmoscope

b. modern diathermy

c. cryotherapy instrumentation

d. soft silicone exoplant/implant materials

e. intraocular gas

8. Which of the following statements about prophylactic therapy is true?

a. Treatment of outer-layer breaks of retinoschisis is valuable.

b. Laser therapy of lattice degeneration is more efficacious than transconjunctival cryotherapy.

c. Prophylactic therapy of lattice degeneration prior to cataract extraction is of proven value.

d. Prophylactic therapy of lattice degeneration associated with atrophic holes is of modest proven value for patients in whom such lesions were associated with retinal detachment in the other eye.

e. Regardless of location, all horseshoe tears should be treated to prevent clinical retinal detachment.

9. The approximate chance of a patient having a problem that can lead to clinical retinal detachment and blindness following the sudden onset of flashes (photopsia) and the sudden appearance of multiple small floating dark "dots" is

a. 0.1%

b. 1%

c. 2%

d. 5%

e. 15%

10. The chance of clinical retinal detachment developing in an eye with lattice degeneration in which atrophic round holes are detected is

a. <0.5%

b. 1%

c. 2.5%

d. 5%

e. 10%

11. The most important visible vitreoretinal precursor of clinical retinal detachment is

a. degenerative retinoschisis

b. atrophic retinal holes

c. lattice degeneration

d. myopic degeneration

e. sex-linked retinoschisis

12. Age-related degenerative retinoschisis

a. commonly extends posteriorly to affect visual acuity

b. is a frequent cause of clinical retinal detachment

c. is usually unilateral

d. usually begins—from a histopathologic standpoint—in the inner plexiform layer

e. none of the above

13. The factor most frequently associated with the development of clinical retinal detachment is

a. a history of cataract extraction

b. a history of blunt trauma

c. diabetes mellitus

d. lattice degeneration

e. a history of penetrating trauma

14. A symptomatic operculated break unassociated with surrounding vitreoretinal traction is less likely to cause clinical retinal detachment than is a symptomatic flap retinal tear associated with persistent vitreoretinal traction (horseshoe tear) by a factor of

a. 2

b. 3

c. 4

d. 5

e. 6

15. The most important vitreoretinal change associated with clinical retinal detachment in patients older than 40 years of age is

a. posterior vitreous detachment

b. lattice degeneration

c. vitreous liquefaction

d. an atrophic retinal break

e. a flap (horseshoe) retinal tear

16. In an eye with a pure traction retinal detachment, the condition least likely to be present is

a. a concave retinal surface

b. sickle cell retinopathy

c. a smooth retinal surface

d. extension of the retinal detachment anterior to the equator

e. vitreous pigment

17. In a patient with a phakic retinal detachment whose visual acuity is 20/20, the one condition most likely to be present is

a. fixed folds

b. large horseshoe tears

c. demarcation lines

d. a macular hole

e. a giant retinal tear

18. The one feature most characteristic of exudative retinal detachments is

a. shifting fluid

b. "tobacco dust"

c. fixed folds

d. equatorial traction folds

e. demarcation lines

19. The vitreoretinal anomaly most likely to lead to retinal detachment is

a. lattice degeneration with atrophic holes

b. a symptomatic operculated tear

c. meridional complex

d. a cystic retinal traction tuft

e. a symptomatic flap tear

20. Which of the following occurs most commonly in association with a retinal detachment in a phakic eye?

a. light flashes

b. vitreous hemorrhage

c. pigmented granules in the vitreous

d. moderate anterior segment cells and flare

e. a history of blunt trauma

ANSWERS AND DISCUSSIONS

1. **Answer—d.** Macular pucker, cystoid macular edema, and subretinal hemorrhage are complications of surgery for retinal detachment that affect postoperative vision. The retinal pigment epithelium frequently exhibits change following chronic detachment of the macula. Pigment "fallout" from cryotherapy is occasionally visible in the macular area. However, pigment granules cannot occupy this position unless the macula has been detached. The relationship between this finding and visual acuity is not completely understood, but reports have demonstrated no apparent effect on postoperative visual acuity.

2. **Answer—b.** Diplopia and refractive errors are common complications of scleral buckling. Subretinal hemorrhage and cataract formation are rare following uneventful retinal surgery. Diffuse preretinal membrane formation (proliferative vitreoretinopathy) is the cause of almost all ultimate anatomic failures.

3. **Answer—d.** Mild ptosis is a common complication of most intraocular surgery. Myopia is a common complication of encircling procedures. Following segmental buckling, astigmatism can occur, particularly if the silicone element is placed anteriorly. Diplopia is a significant complication of scleral buckling. Hyperopia, however, is usually not observed in association with surgery for retinal detachment.

4. **Answer—d.** Eyes with retinal detachments that involve the macula generally have a poor visual outcome compared to those without macular involvement. Although there are exceptions, the duration of macular detachment tends to be inversely related to postoperative visual acuity. Preoperative visual acuity has been demonstrated in many studies as the factor most predictive of visual outcome following successful retinal reattachment surgery.

5. **Answer—b.** Choroidal detachments rarely affect anatomic success. Recurrent retinal detachments due to new breaks, "inadequate" scleral buckles, or "inadequate" chorioretinal adhesions can usually be repaired unless they are associated with the development of diffuse epiretinal membranes (proliferative vitreoretinopathy). Proliferative vitreoretinopathy is responsible for virtually all ultimate anatomic failures following retinal detachment surgery.

6. **Answer—c.** Since the time of Gonin, a wide range of visual acuity has been observed following successful surgery for retinal detachment. Despite dramatic improvements in anatomic success rates, visual successes have not improved significantly over the past few decades.

7. **Answer—a.** The recognition and localization of significant retinal breaks remain the most important factors in successful surgery for retinal detachment. Once discovered, such breaks can be managed in a variety of ways. The binocular indirect ophthalmoscope, developed by Schepens, provides a stereoscopic image of relatively large areas of the retina. The production of this instrument has been the most important advance in retinal surgery since the work of Gonin.

8. **Answer—d.** Prophylactic therapy for breaks in retinoschisis and for asymptomatic horseshoe tears in eyes without high-risk features has been demonstrated to be of no apparent value. Prophylactic therapy of lattice degeneration prior to cataract extraction is not of proven value. Laser therapy and transconjunctival cryotherapy may be of equal value in treating selected cases of lattice degeneration. Studies have demonstrated a modest benefit from treating lattice degeneration in the fellow eye of patients who have had a previous retinal detachment associated with lattice degeneration in the other eye.

9. **Answer—e.** Multiple studies have demonstrated that approximately 15% of eyes with symptoms of posterior vitreous detachment and modest vitreous hemorrhage will have associated retinal breaks.

10. **Answer—a.** Lattice degeneration occurs in approximately 8% of the population, but most retinal detachments associated with lattice degeneration are due to horseshoe tears. Atrophic round holes in lattice degeneration cause retinal detachments in relatively young patients with myopia, and they typically occur prior to complete posterior vitreous detachment. In most retinal detachments, however, atrophic round holes are rarely the cause of the detachment.

11. **Answer—c.** Degenerative retinoschisis is an unusual cause of clinical rhegmatogenous retinal detachment, and atrophic retinal holes unassociated with lattice degeneration are a rare cause of this problem. Retinal detachments associated with sex-linked retinoschisis are unusual, and "myopic degeneration" is not a recognized cause of retinal detachment (although retinal detachment is much more common in myopic eyes). Lattice degeneration is observed in approximately one third of cases with rhegmatogenous retinal detachment.

12. **Answer—e.** Age-related degenerative retinoschisis is believed to be a continuum of confluent peripheral cystoid degeneration, beginning in the outer plexiform layer. It is usually bilateral and is an unusual cause of clinical retinal detachment. It rarely extends to affect macular function.

13. **Answer—a.** Although frequently associated with rhegmatogenous retinal detachment, lattice degeneration occurs in only 8% of the population, and within this 8% retinal detachments are relatively unusual. Diabetes mellitus is an important cause of traction and combined retinal detachments. Blunt and penetrating traumas are significant causes of retinal detachment. However, as many as 40% of retinal detachment cases referred for surgery have a history of cataract extraction.

14. **Answer—e.** Operculated retinal breaks unassociated with persistent vitreous traction on the surrounding retina are a rare cause of clinical retinal detachment, whereas symptomatic horseshoe tears commonly progress to detachment.

15. **Answer—a.** Atrophic retinal breaks are an uncommon cause of clinical retinal detachment. Vitreous liquefaction occurs in all adults. Lattice degeneration and horseshoe tears of the retina are significant causes of clinical retinal detachment. However, posterior vitreous detachment with subsequent vitreoretinal traction on sites of vitreoretinal adhesion is the most important change leading to clinical rhegmatogenous retinal detachment.

16. **Answer—e.** Pigmented granules are almost pathognomonic of a retinal tear of retinal detachment in an eye that has never had intraocular surgery. Most traction retinal detachments do not extend to the ora serrata, although they may extend relatively anteriorly. The other findings are characteristic of those associated with traction retinal detachment.

17. **Answer—c.** Retinal detachments with fixed folds, giant retinal tears, and large horseshoe tears usually progress rapidly to cause macular detachment and diminished visual acuity. Long-standing retinal detachments represent a major exception. Many patients with long-standing detachments have demarcation lines and normal visual acuity. A corrugated appearance of the retina usually implies recent retinal detachment.

18. **Answer—a.** Shifting fluid is a hallmark finding of exudative retinal detachment, although it may occasionally be seen in the rhegmatogenous variety, particularly following cataract surgery. All the other findings are very characteristic of rhegmatogenous retinal detachment.

19. **Answer—e.** Symptomatic horseshoe (flap) tears progress to clinical retinal detachment in approximately 50% of cases. Lattice degeneration with atrophic holes and cystic retinal traction tufts may be associated with retinal detachments, but they are much less significant. Symptomatic operculated breaks unassociated with surrounding vitreoretinal traction are an uncommon cause of clinical retinal detachment. Of the vitreoretinal anomalies listed, meridional complexes are least likely to cause clinical retinal detachment.

20. **Answer—c.** Pigmented granules are usually indicative of a retinal tear or retinal detachment in an eye that has never had intraocular surgery. All of the other findings may be observed in eyes with posterior vitreous detachments, retinal tear formation, and retinal detachment, but many patients have these problems without an associated significant retinal break.

INDEX

NOTE: An *f* following a page number indicates a figure, and a *t* following a page number indicates a table. Drugs are usually listed under their generic names; when a drug trade name is listed, the reader is referred to the generic name.

I

J

K

S